HISTAMINE INTOLERANCE COOKBOOK

The Complete 14-Day Diet Meal Plan With Delicious And Nourishing Recipes For Healthy Living.

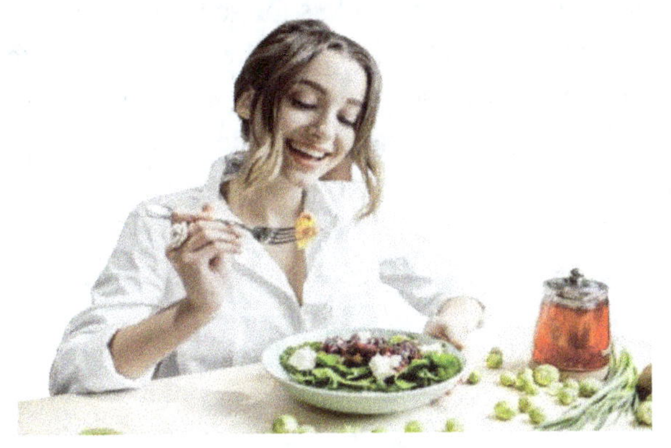

AVELINE WINTER

TABLE OF CONTENT

INTRODUCTION

Welcome to a journey of flavorful nourishment designed specifically for those managing histamine intolerance. This cookbook aims to revolutionize your culinary experience by providing a diverse array of delectable dishes while ensuring they adhere to a low histamine diet.

Living with histamine intolerance can present challenges, but this cookbook aims to transform those challenges into opportunities for creativity and wellness. From comforting breakfasts to satisfying dinners, each recipe has been meticulously crafted to cater to your dietary needs without compromising on taste or nutrition.

Within these pages, you'll discover a meticulously curated 14-day meal plan, offering a variety of dishes infused with low histamine ingredients. Embrace the abundance of fresh produce, lean proteins, and alternative grains as you embark on this flavorful journey.

We've included detailed guidance on ingredient selection, cooking methods that preserve low histamine levels, portion sizes for balanced nutrient intake, and tips for handling and storing foods to reduce histamine buildup. Moreover, we offer substitutions to accommodate various dietary needs, ensuring this meal plan is adaptable for everyone.

It's essential to note that individual tolerance levels can vary. This meal plan serves as a guideline, but listening to your body's response to different foods is key. Let this cookbook be your companion on a delicious and healthful journey toward managing histamine intolerance. Enjoy the flavors, savor the variety, and relish the satisfaction of nurturing your body with these thoughtfully crafted, low histamine recipes.

Bon Appétit and here's to a journey of culinary delight and wellness!

Understanding Histamine Intolerance

Histamine intolerance refers to a condition where the body has difficulty metabolizing histamine effectively. Histamine is a natural compound produced by the body and is also found in certain foods. It plays a crucial role in the immune system, acting as a signaling molecule involved in various bodily functions.

Causes:
The underlying cause of histamine intolerance often involves a deficiency in the enzyme diamine oxidase (DAO) or histamine N-methyltransferase (HNMT), responsible for breaking down histamine. When these enzymes are insufficient, the body struggles to process excess histamine efficiently, leading to an accumulation in the bloodstream.

Effects on the Body:
When histamine levels rise due to inefficient breakdown, it can trigger various symptoms, including but not limited to:
- Skin reactions like hives or rashes
- Headaches or migraines
- Digestive issues such as abdominal pain, bloating, or diarrhea
- Respiratory problems like nasal congestion or difficulty breathing
- Irregular heart rate or blood pressure fluctuations

Histamine intolerance doesn't involve an allergic reaction but rather a sensitivity to histamine. Certain factors can exacerbate this sensitivity, such as consuming foods high in histamine, certain medications, alcohol, or stress.

Metabolism Challenges:
In individuals with histamine intolerance, the body's inability to break down histamine efficiently leads to an accumulation of this compound. This occurs particularly when consuming foods high in histamine or substances that trigger the body to release histamine.

Management:
Managing histamine intolerance involves adopting a low histamine diet, which focuses on avoiding high histamine foods and opting for fresh, minimally processed options. It often requires careful attention to food choices, labels, and cooking methods to reduce histamine intake. Additionally,

stress management and lifestyle adjustments can also play a role in managing symptoms.

Seeking guidance from healthcare professionals or dietitians can aid in developing a personalized approach to managing histamine intolerance, ensuring individuals can enjoy a better quality of life by minimizing histamine-triggered symptoms.

Symptoms and Triggers

Common Symptoms:
Histamine intolerance can manifest through a range of symptoms that vary in severity and presentation among individuals. Some common symptoms include:

1. Headaches or Migraines: Histamine can dilate blood vessels, leading to headaches or migraines in sensitive individuals.

2. Skin Reactions: Rashes, hives, or itching can occur due to increased histamine levels affecting the skin's blood vessels and immune response.

3. Digestive Issues: Abdominal pain, bloating, diarrhea, or constipation may arise due to histamine's influence on gut motility and function.

4. Respiratory Problems: Nasal congestion, sneezing, coughing, or difficulty breathing can be triggered by histamine, impacting the respiratory system.

5. Cardiovascular Symptoms: Histamine can influence blood pressure and heart rate, leading to irregularities or fluctuations in sensitive individuals.

Potential Triggers:
Several factors can trigger or exacerbate histamine intolerance symptoms. Common triggers include:

1. Histamine-Rich Foods: Certain foods are naturally high in histamine or can trigger the release of histamine in the body. Examples include aged cheeses, fermented foods, processed meats, and some vegetables (like tomatoes).

2. Alcohol: Especially red wine and beer contain histamine and can prompt the body to release more histamine, triggering symptoms in sensitive individuals.

3. Environmental Factors: Pollen, dust mites, pet dander, or other environmental allergens can stimulate histamine production or worsen symptoms in those with histamine intolerance.

4. Medications: Some medications, particularly certain pain relievers, antibiotics, and medications used for stomach acid control, can interfere with histamine breakdown or trigger histamine release.

5. Stress: Emotional or physical stress can exacerbate symptoms by affecting the body's ability to regulate histamine levels.

Recognizing these symptoms and triggers can help individuals identify and manage their histamine intolerance more effectively. It's essential to maintain a diary to track food intake, environmental exposures, and symptoms to identify specific triggers unique to you.

Low Histamine Diet Essentials

A low histamine diet is a fundamental approach for managing histamine intolerance. It revolves around choosing foods that are less likely to trigger histamine release or contain lower levels of histamine, emphasizing fresh, minimally processed options. The key principles include:

1. Fresh and Minimally Processed Foods:
  - Opt for fresh, unprocessed foods whenever possible. Fresh fruits, vegetables, lean meats, and freshly caught fish are generally lower in histamine.
  - Choose fresh cuts of meat, poultry, and fish rather than processed or cured varieties that tend to have higher histamine levels.

2. Avoidance of High Histamine Foods:

- Foods known to be high in histamine should be avoided or minimized. These include aged or fermented products like aged cheeses, cured meats, sauerkraut, soy sauce, and certain pickled foods.

- Additionally, leftovers or foods that have been stored for a prolonged period can accumulate higher levels of histamine, so consuming freshly prepared meals is advisable.

3. Fresh Dairy Alternatives:

- Dairy products can be high in histamine, so opting for fresh, pasteurized milk, or low histamine alternatives like rice milk, hemp milk, or oat milk can be beneficial.

4. Careful Selection of Fruits and Vegetables:

- While most fruits and vegetables are well-tolerated, some individuals may find that certain varieties trigger symptoms. Opt for fresh produce and be mindful of personal tolerances.

- Cooking fruits and vegetables can sometimes lower their histamine content, making them more tolerable for some individuals.

5. Mindful Grain Choices:

- Grains like wheat can be problematic for some due to potential mold content. Opting for gluten-free alternatives like rice, quinoa, or millet might be more suitable for those sensitive to histamine.

6. Attention to Food Additives and Preservatives:

- Artificial additives, colorings, and preservatives commonly found in processed foods can trigger histamine release or interfere with histamine breakdown. Reading labels and avoiding these additives is recommended.

7. Fresh Herbs and Spices:

- While some spices can be high in histamine, fresh herbs and selected spices might be better tolerated. Experimenting with fresh herbs like basil, parsley, or thyme can add flavor without triggering symptoms.

Adopting a low histamine diet involves mindful food selection, meal preparation, and being attentive to individual responses to different foods. Keeping a food diary to track intake and associated symptoms can help identify trigger foods unique to each person.

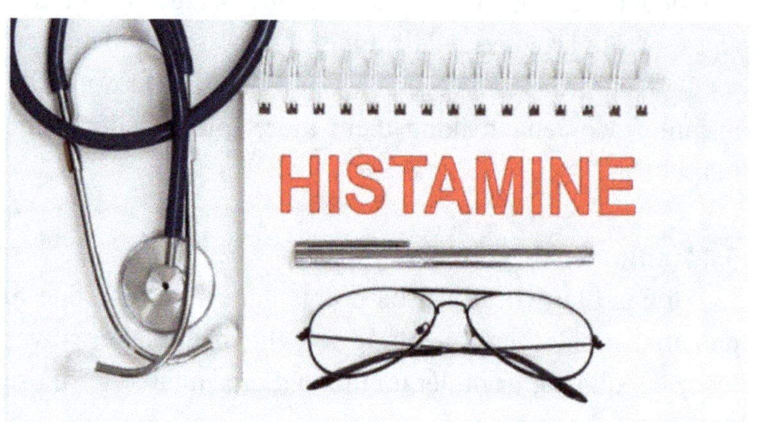

Reading Food Labels for Histamine Intolerance:

Understanding how to read food labels is crucial for individuals managing histamine intolerance. Here are some tips to identify and avoid high histamine ingredients or additives:

1. Check for Histamine-Rich Ingredients:
  - Look for common high histamine ingredients such as:
  - Aged or fermented foods: Including aged cheeses (cheddar, blue cheese), fermented soy products (soy sauce, miso), and pickled items.
  - Cured or processed meats: Salami, pepperoni, and other processed meats often contain higher levels of histamine.
  - Vinegar or alcohol: Certain types of vinegar (especially red wine vinegar) and alcoholic beverages can be high in histamine.

2. Watch for Food Additives and Preservatives:
  - Certain food additives and preservatives can trigger histamine release or interfere with histamine breakdown. Avoid ingredients like:
  - Artificial colorings and flavorings: Look out for terms like "artificial color," "artificial flavor," or specific color numbers.
  - Sulfites and sulfates: Commonly found in dried fruits, preserved vegetables, and processed meats, these can

provoke histamine-related symptoms in sensitive individuals.

3. Mind the 'Use By' or 'Best Before' Dates:

- Foods that have been stored for an extended period may have higher histamine levels. Choose fresh products with dates further from expiration.

4. Choose Fresh and Whole Foods:

- Opt for whole, fresh foods whenever possible. Fresh fruits, vegetables, and meats are generally lower in histamine than their processed counterparts.

5. Be Cautious with Packaged and Processed Foods:

- Processed and ready-to-eat meals often contain hidden sources of histamine. Check ingredient lists carefully and prefer homemade or freshly prepared meals.

6. Read Ingredient Lists Carefully:

- Scan ingredient lists for any mention of high histamine ingredients or additives. These might not always be obvious, so being thorough is important.

7. Stay Informed and Updated:

- Stay informed about potential high histamine ingredients or additives by researching and keeping up-to-date with reliable sources and reputable information.

Understanding food labels is a key aspect of managing histamine intolerance. By being vigilant about ingredients and additives that may trigger symptoms, you can make informed choices to minimize their exposure to high histamine foods.

Cooking Techniques for Histamine Intolerance

Cooking methods play a pivotal role in managing histamine levels in food while ensuring nutrient retention. Here are some preferred techniques that minimize histamine accumulation:

1. Grilling:
  - Grilling is a favorable method as it allows excess fats and juices to drip away from the food, reducing the potential for histamine formation.
  - It's ideal for cooking meats, fish, and vegetables. However, be cautious with prolonged marination or using high histamine sauces or spices in grilling preparations.

2. Baking or Roasting:
  - Baking or roasting food in the oven at moderate temperatures can help preserve nutrients while minimizing histamine formation.
  - Choose fresh cuts of meat, poultry, or fish, and avoid using high histamine ingredients or long marination times before baking.

3. Steaming:

- Steaming is a gentle cooking method that retains moisture and nutrients in foods without causing histamine buildup.

- It's especially suitable for vegetables, fish, and poultry. Steaming vegetables lightly can also make them easier to digest for sensitive individuals.

4. Boiling:

- Boiling is effective for cooking grains, legumes, and some vegetables. It can reduce histamine levels, but be cautious not to overcook, which may lead to nutrient loss.

- Use fresh ingredients and avoid prolonged boiling times to minimize histamine accumulation.

5. Blanching:

- Blanching involves briefly immersing vegetables or fruits in boiling water, then quickly cooling them in ice water. This method can reduce histamine levels while maintaining texture and color.

- It's particularly useful for preparing vegetables before freezing or for making salads.

6. Avoid Fermentation and Prolonged Storage:

- Fermentation processes, like in pickling or fermenting foods, can significantly increase histamine levels. Avoid such techniques in meal preparation.

- Opt for fresh ingredients and minimize leftovers or foods stored for extended periods, as they tend to accumulate histamine.

7. Prefer Fresh Ingredients:
   - Using fresh, minimally processed ingredients is crucial. Fresh fruits, vegetables, meats, and fish are generally lower in histamine than their processed counterparts.

Understanding these cooking techniques empowers individuals managing histamine intolerance to prepare meals that are lower in histamine while retaining vital nutrients. Experimenting with these methods can help in crafting delicious and nourishing dishes suitable for a low histamine diet.

Foods High in Histamine You Should Avoid

1. Aged Cheeses:
   - Aged cheeses like Parmesan, Gouda, Cheddar, and Blue cheese contain higher levels of histamine due to the fermentation process. Consider opting for fresh cheeses like mozzarella or cottage cheese.

2. Fermented Foods:
   - Fermented foods such as sauerkraut, kimchi, pickles, and soy-based products like miso or soy sauce can have elevated histamine levels.

3. Processed Meats:
   - Processed meats including salami, pepperoni, bacon, and sausages often have higher histamine content compared to

freshly prepared meats. Fresh cuts of meat are generally better tolerated.

4. Certain Seafoods:

- Certain types of seafood, particularly shellfish like shrimp, lobster, and crab, can contain higher levels of histamine, especially when not fresh.

5. Alcohol:

- Alcoholic beverages, especially red wine, beer, and champagne, can provoke histamine release and interfere with histamine breakdown.

6. Vinegar and Fermented Condiments:

- Foods with high vinegar content like ketchup, mustard, mayonnaise, and salad dressings, as well as fermented condiments, can contribute to higher histamine levels.

7. Certain Fruits and Vegetables:

- Histamine levels in fruits and vegetables can vary. Some individuals may be sensitive to avocados, tomatoes, spinach, eggplants, and citrus fruits like oranges or lemons.

8. Dried Fruits and Nuts:

- Dried fruits and nuts can have increased histamine levels due to the drying process. Opt for fresh fruits and limit intake of dried varieties.

9. Canned or Smoked Fish:

- Canned or smoked fish, such as canned tuna or smoked salmon, may have higher histamine content compared to freshly cooked fish.

10. Certain Grains and Legumes:

- Some grains and legumes, especially those that have been stored for a prolonged period, may contain higher histamine levels. Examples include chickpeas, lentils, and some types of rice.

11. Chocolate and Cocoa Products:

- Chocolate and cocoa products can contain histamine and other compounds that may trigger symptoms in sensitive individuals.

12. Food Additives and Preservatives:

- Artificial additives, colorings, and preservatives commonly found in processed foods can contribute to histamine release or interfere with histamine breakdown.

Avoiding or reducing intake of these high histamine foods may help individuals manage their histamine intolerance and minimize the risk of triggering histamine-related symptoms.

Managing Histamine Levels:

Managing histamine levels involves not only dietary considerations but also lifestyle adjustments and stress reduction techniques. Here are some tips:

1. Stress Management:

- Stress can exacerbate histamine intolerance symptoms. Engage in stress-relieving activities such as meditation, yoga, deep breathing exercises, or mindfulness practices.

- Prioritize adequate sleep and establish a consistent sleep schedule to reduce stress levels and promote overall well-being.

2. Regular Exercise:

- Engaging in regular physical activity can help regulate histamine levels and improve overall health. Opt for activities like walking, swimming, or gentle yoga to avoid excessive stress on the body.

3. Allergen Control:

- Reduce exposure to environmental allergens such as pollen, dust mites, or pet dander, which can trigger histamine release.

- Use air purifiers or take measures to keep living spaces clean and free from potential allergens.

4. Temperature and Weather Consideration:

- Extreme temperatures, especially heat, can stimulate histamine release. Stay cool in warmer weather and dress appropriately to minimize reactions.

5. Hydration and Detoxification:

- Staying hydrated supports the body's detoxification processes, aiding in histamine clearance. Consume adequate water and herbal teas throughout the day.
- Consider incorporating foods that support liver health, such as cruciferous vegetables (broccoli, kale), which may assist in histamine metabolism.

6. Supplementation and Medications:

- Consult healthcare professionals about potential supplements or medications that may help manage histamine levels. Some individuals find relief with specific supplements, but it's essential to seek guidance before taking any.

7. Mindfulness and Self-Care:

- Practice self-awareness and mindfulness about your body's responses to different environments, foods, or situations.
- Prioritize self-care routines that promote relaxation and well-being, such as aromatherapy, massage, or taking time for hobbies and interests.

8. Seek Professional Guidance:

- Consult with healthcare providers or specialists knowledgeable about histamine intolerance. They can provide personalized advice and guidance tailored to your specific needs.

By incorporating these lifestyle adjustments and stress reduction techniques into daily routines, individuals managing histamine intolerance can complement their dietary efforts and potentially reduce the frequency and severity of symptoms associated with histamine reactions.

Individual Variability

Histamine intolerance manifests uniquely in each individual, varying in severity, symptoms, and tolerance levels. Understanding this variability is essential for managing histamine intolerance effectively.

1. Symptom Variations:

- Individuals with histamine intolerance can experience a wide range of symptoms. Some may have mild reactions like slight headaches or occasional digestive discomfort, while others may experience more pronounced symptoms such as severe migraines, skin rashes, or respiratory issues.

2. Tolerance Levels:

- Tolerance levels for histamine-rich foods or triggers vary significantly among individuals. One person might be highly sensitive to certain foods, while another might tolerate them in moderation without adverse effects.

3. Factors Influencing Variability:

- Genetic factors, the degree of enzyme deficiency (such as DAO or HNMT), overall health status, gut health, and individual immune responses all contribute to the variability in histamine intolerance.

4. Personalized Triggers:

- Certain individuals may have specific triggers unique to them. While common high histamine foods exist, personal tolerance levels can differ. It's crucial for each person to identify their individual triggers through observation and possibly keeping a food diary.

5. Response to Environmental Factors:

- Environmental factors, stress levels, lifestyle, and overall health can influence how the body reacts to histamine. Some may find that stress exacerbates symptoms, while others might notice no significant impact.

6. Gradual Introduction and Observation:

- It's essential for individuals managing histamine intolerance to gradually introduce new foods into their diet, observing how their bodies respond. This approach helps identify personal tolerances and triggers.

7. Professional Guidance and Self-Awareness:

- Seeking guidance from healthcare professionals or dietitians specializing in histamine intolerance can assist in understanding individual variability. They can help create personalized plans considering unique sensitivities.

- Practicing self-awareness and mindfulness about one's body and its responses to various foods, environments, or situations is crucial in managing histamine intolerance effectively.

Understanding the individual variability associated with histamine intolerance empowers individuals to tailor their dietary and lifestyle choices to their unique needs. By being attentive to personal triggers and tolerance levels, individuals can better manage their condition and minimize the impact of histamine-related symptoms.

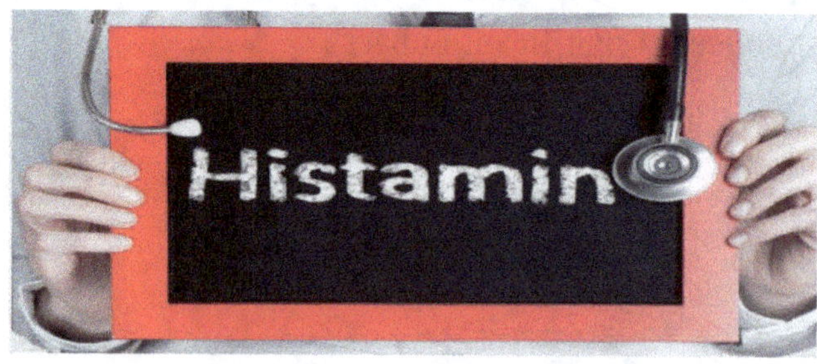

14-Day Low Histamine Meal

Welcome to Your 14-Day Low Histamine Meal Adventure!

Hey there! Ready to embark on a flavorful journey that's not just about eating but about feeling your absolute best? Welcome to your 14-day low histamine meal plan – your ticket to savoring delicious meals while giving your body the TLC it deserves.

Why Low Histamine, You Ask?

Well, histamine intolerance is like that uninvited guest at the party – it shows up when you least expect it. But fear not, this meal plan is here to help you manage it like a pro! Histamine intolerance can cause a bit of a ruckus in our bodies, but with the right foods and a touch of culinary creativity, we can keep those pesky symptoms at bay.

Deliciousness Awaits!

We've crafted this meal plan with one thing in mind: flavor without the fuss. Expect a smorgasbord of delectable dishes that not only tantalize your taste buds but also adhere to low histamine principles. From comforting breakfasts to satisfying dinners, each meal is a celebration of fresh, wholesome ingredients that your body will love.

More Than Just Recipes

But hey, this isn't just about recipes – it's a guide to help you navigate the maze of histamine intolerance. We've packed it with tips on ingredient selection, cooking methods that keep histamine levels in check, and even strategies for handling and storing foods to keep those histamine levels down.

Your Journey, Your Pace

Remember, this isn't a one-size-fits-all journey. Listen to your body, savor each bite, and take note of what works best for you. Consider this meal plan as your friendly GPS – guiding you, but ultimately, you're in the driver's seat.

So, here's to indulging in mouthwatering meals, to nurturing your body, and to feeling fantastic every step of the way. Get ready to dive in and relish these next 14 days of flavorful adventures!

Bon Appétit and let's make these 14 days simply delicious and nourishing!

WEEK 1

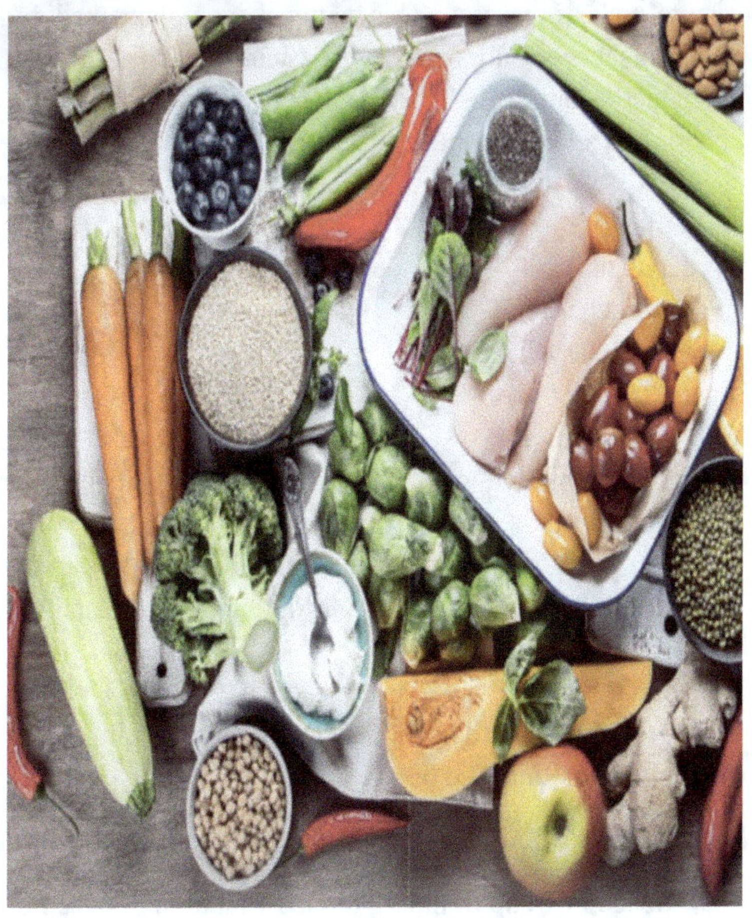

Day 1

- Breakfast: Blueberry Oatmeal Energizer

Introduction: Morning routines call for a nourishing yet easy-to-make breakfast. This oatmeal, complemented by fresh blueberries and a touch of pasteurized milk, offers a deliciously comforting way to kickstart your day while adhering to a low histamine diet.

Ingredients:
- ½ cup Oats
- Fresh blueberries
- Splash of pasteurized milk

Cooking Method:
Step 1: Combine ½ cup of oats with 1 cup of water or pasteurized milk in a saucepan.
Step 2: Cook the mixture over medium heat, stirring occasionally, until the oats absorb the liquid and reach the desired consistency.
Step 3: Transfer the cooked oatmeal to a bowl.
Step 4: Garnish the oatmeal generously with fresh blueberries for an added burst of flavor.

Portion Sizes: For a balanced serving, aim for ½ cup of dry oats cooked in 1 cup of liquid, topped with around ½ cup of fresh blueberries.

Storage and Handling Tips: Store oats in an airtight container in a cool, dry place. Keep fresh blueberries refrigerated and consume them within a few days for optimal taste and nutritional benefits.

Substitutions: Replace pasteurized milk with dairy-free alternatives like almond or coconut milk for those with dairy sensitivities. Gluten-free oats can be used for individuals following a gluten-free diet.

Hydration and Beverages: Complement this nutritious oatmeal breakfast with a glass of water, herbal tea, or a suitable fruit juice (avoiding citrus) to ensure adequate hydration.

Individual Tolerance: Always be mindful of individual tolerance levels. Monitor how your body responds to oats, blueberries, and milk alternatives, adjusting portion sizes accordingly to suit your dietary needs without triggering adverse reactions.

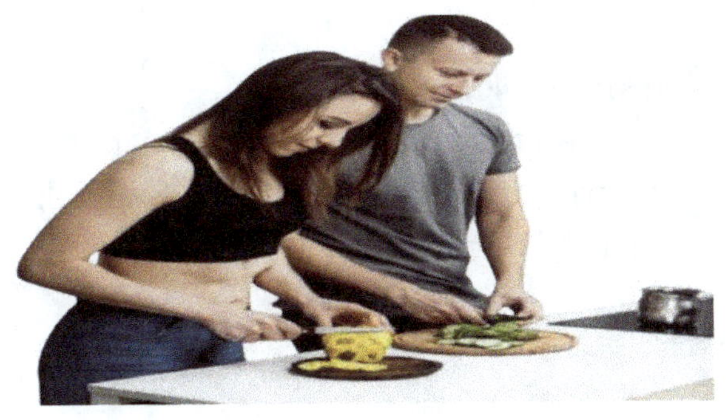

- Lunch: Grilled Chicken Lunch Delight

Introduction: For a satisfying midday meal that's both flavorful and histamine-friendly, this grilled chicken dish paired with steamed asparagus and boiled sweet potatoes hits the spot. It's a well-balanced plate that's gentle on a low histamine diet.

Ingredients:
- Chicken breast
- Asparagus
- Sweet potatoes
- Seasonings (salt, pepper, herbs - low histamine options)

Cooking Method:
Step 1 - Grilled Chicken:
- Preheat the grill to medium-high heat.
- Season the chicken breast with salt, pepper, and preferred low histamine herbs.
- Grill the chicken for about 6-8 minutes per side or until fully cooked through.

Step 2 - Steamed Asparagus:
- Trim the woody ends off the asparagus spears.
- Steam the asparagus in a steamer basket over boiling water for approximately 3-5 minutes until tender but still crisp.

Step 3 - Boiled Sweet Potatoes:
- Peel and dice the sweet potatoes into cubes.
- Boil the sweet potato cubes in a pot of water until fork-tender, usually around 10-15 minutes.

Portion Sizes: Aim for a palm-sized portion of grilled chicken, about 5-6 asparagus spears, and half to one small sweet potato for a well-rounded meal.

Storage and Handling Tips: Store raw chicken separately in the refrigerator to prevent cross-contamination. Asparagus should be refrigerated and consumed within a few days, while sweet potatoes can be stored in a cool, dark place.

Substitutions: Tofu or tempeh can be used as vegetarian substitutes for chicken. For vegan options, swap chicken with grilled portobello mushrooms. Various herbs like basil, thyme, or oregano can be used for seasoning.

Hydration and Beverages: Accompany this lunch with water, herbal teas, or suitable fruit juices (avoiding citrus) to support hydration throughout the day.

Individual Tolerance: Remember, individual tolerance levels can vary. Observe your body's response to these ingredients and adjust portion sizes or make ingredient substitutions if needed to suit your specific needs.

- Dinner: Baked Fish and Sautéed Broccoli Delight

Introduction: A nutritious yet histamine-friendly dinner option awaits with this baked fish served alongside sautéed broccoli. This meal keeps things simple, flavorful, and suitable for those adhering to a low histamine diet.

Ingredients:
- Fresh or frozen fish filets (low histamine options)
- Broccoli
- Animal fats (e.g., butter or ghee)
- Seasonings (salt, pepper, herbs - low histamine options)

Cooking Method:
Step 1 - Baked Fish:
- Preheat the oven to 375°F (190°C).
- Place the fish filets on a baking sheet lined with parchment paper.
- Season the fish with salt, pepper, and preferred low histamine herbs.
- Bake the fish for about 15-20 minutes or until it flakes easily with a fork.

Step 2 - Sautéed Broccoli:
- Cut the broccoli into florets.
- Heat animal fats (such as butter or ghee) in a pan over medium heat.
- Add the broccoli florets to the pan and sauté for about 5-7 minutes until tender yet crisp.

Portion Sizes: A suitable portion of fish is typically around 3-6 ounces per serving, while 1-2 cups of sautéed broccoli makes a balanced side dish.

Storage and Handling Tips: Store fish in the refrigerator and use within a few days. Broccoli should be kept refrigerated in a sealed container and consumed within a week for optimal freshness.

Substitutions: For vegetarian or vegan options, replace fish with tofu or tempeh baked with similar seasonings. Substitute animal fats with olive oil or coconut oil for a dairy-free alternative.

Hydration and Beverages: Enjoy this meal with a glass of water, herbal tea, or a suitable fruit juice (avoiding citrus) to ensure proper hydration.

Individual Tolerance: Always be attentive to your body's reactions to different foods. Adjust portion sizes and ingredients as needed to align with your dietary needs and avoid triggering histamine reactions.

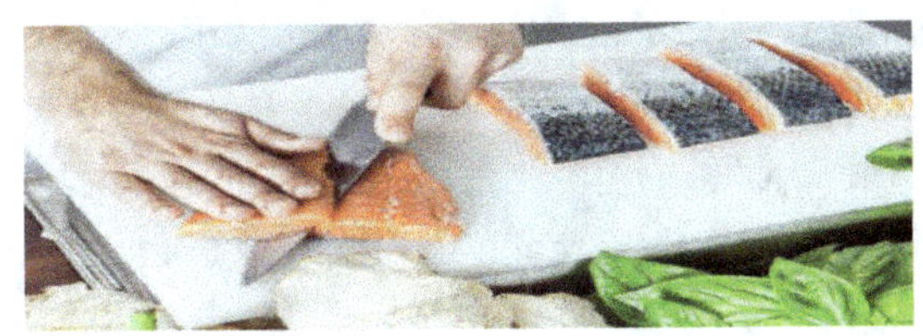

Day 2

- Breakfast: Scrumptious Scrambled Eggs Delight

Introduction: Start your day on a savory note with this delectable breakfast featuring scrambled eggs enriched with sautéed onions and fresh herbs. This dish not only tantalizes your taste buds but also aligns perfectly with a low histamine diet.

Ingredients:
- Eggs (yolks only)
- Onions
- Fresh herbs (low histamine options)
- Cooking oil or animal fats
- Seasonings (salt, pepper)

Cooking Method:
Step 1 - Scrambled Eggs:
- Crack eggs and separate the yolks from the whites. Use only the yolks.
- Whisk the yolks gently in a bowl and season with salt and pepper.
- Heat cooking oil or animal fats in a skillet over medium heat.
- Pour the yolks into the skillet and cook, stirring continuously, until they reach the desired consistency.

Step 2 - Sautéed Onions and Fresh Herbs:
- Thinly slice the onions and chop the fresh herbs.
- Heat a little cooking oil or animal fats in a separate pan over medium heat.
- Sauté the onions until they turn translucent and slightly golden.
- Add the fresh herbs and cook for an additional minute, stirring gently.

Portion Sizes: For a balanced breakfast, aim for 2-3 egg yolks per serving, along with a quarter to half a cup of sautéed onions and a sprinkle of fresh herbs.

Storage and Handling Tips: Store eggs in the refrigerator and use them within a reasonable time. Onions and fresh herbs should be stored in a cool, dry place or the refrigerator to maintain their freshness.

Substitutions: For a vegan alternative, consider using scrambled tofu instead of eggs. Replace animal fats with plant-based oils like olive oil or coconut oil.

Hydration and Beverages: Pair this savory breakfast with water, herbal teas, or suitable fruit juices (avoiding citrus) to ensure proper hydration throughout the morning.

Individual Tolerance: As individual tolerance levels can vary, monitor your body's response to different foods. Adjust portion sizes or make ingredient substitutions as necessary to suit your specific dietary needs without triggering adverse reactions.

- Lunch: Vibrant Rice Bowl Medley

Introduction: Enjoy a colorful and nutritious lunch with this delightful rice bowl. Packed with cooked beets, refreshing cucumber slices, and savory grilled chicken, this dish offers a satisfying yet histamine-friendly option for your midday meal.

Ingredients:
- Cooked rice (low histamine grain)
- Beets
- Cucumber
- Grilled chicken (or alternative protein)
- Seasonings (salt, pepper, herbs - low histamine options)

Cooking Method:
Step 1 - Cooked Rice:
- Prepare the rice according to package instructions using your preferred low histamine grain. Set aside.

Step 2 - Cooked Beets:
- Peel and dice the beets into cubes.
- Boil or steam the beet cubes until they are fork-tender, usually for about 15-20 minutes.

Step 3 - Cucumber Slices:
- Wash and slice the cucumber into thin rounds.

Step 4 - Grilled Chicken (or alternative protein):
- Season the chicken with salt, pepper, and preferred low histamine herbs.
- Grill the chicken for about 6-8 minutes per side or until fully cooked through.
- Alternatively, prepare your choice of alternative protein according to your dietary preferences.

Portion Sizes: Aim for a balanced bowl with around 1 cup of cooked rice, a quarter to a half cup of cooked beets, a handful of cucumber slices, and a palm-sized portion of grilled chicken or alternative protein.

Storage and Handling Tips: Store leftover cooked rice and beets in airtight containers in the refrigerator for up to 3-4 days. Cucumbers should be kept refrigerated and consumed within a few days.

Substitutions: Replace grilled chicken with tofu, tempeh, or legumes for vegetarian or vegan options. Consider using quinoa or other low histamine grains as an alternative to rice.

Hydration and Beverages: Pair this vibrant rice bowl with water, herbal teas, or suitable fruit juices (avoiding citrus) to maintain proper hydration levels throughout the day.

Individual Tolerance: Always be mindful of individual reactions to different foods. Adjust portion sizes or make ingredient substitutions as needed to align with your specific dietary needs and avoid triggering histamine reactions.

- Dinner: Bountiful Baked Salmon Feast

Introduction: Indulge in a flavorful and nourishing dinner featuring baked salmon accompanied by creamy mashed potatoes and delicate steamed squash. This wholesome meal caters to a low histamine diet while offering a delightful dining experience.

Ingredients:
- Salmon filets (fresh or frozen)
- Potatoes
- Squash
- Seasonings (salt, pepper, herbs - low histamine options)
- Butter or dairy-free alternative (for mashed potatoes)

Cooking Method:
Step 1 - Baked Salmon:
- Preheat the oven to 375°F (190°C).
- Season the salmon filets with salt, pepper, and preferred low histamine herbs.
- Place the seasoned salmon on a baking sheet lined with parchment paper.
- Bake the salmon for approximately 12-15 minutes until it flakes easily with a fork.

Step 2 - Mashed Potatoes:
- Peel and chop the potatoes into chunks.
- Boil the potato chunks in salted water until they are tender, usually for about 15-20 minutes.
- Drain the potatoes and mash them using butter or a dairy-free alternative. Season to taste.

Step 3 - Steamed Squash:
- Cut the squash into slices or cubes.
- Steam the squash in a steamer basket over boiling water for about 5-7 minutes until it's tender but not mushy.

Portion Sizes: Aim for a balanced meal with a palm-sized portion of salmon, about 1 cup of mashed potatoes, and a portion of steamed squash that suits your preference.

Storage and Handling Tips: Store any leftover salmon, mashed potatoes, and squash in airtight containers in the refrigerator. Consume within 2-3 days for optimal taste and freshness.

Substitutions: Substitute salmon with another low histamine fish or tofu for vegetarian or vegan options. For dairy-free mashed potatoes, use plant-based butter or olive oil.

Hydration and Beverages: Complement this delightful dinner with water, herbal teas, or suitable fruit juices (avoiding citrus) to maintain adequate hydration.

Individual Tolerance: Keep track of how your body responds to different foods. Adjust portion sizes or make ingredient substitutions as needed to accommodate your specific dietary needs and prevent histamine reactions.

Day 3

- Breakfast: Exquisite Fresh Fruit Morning Delight

Introduction: Elevate your mornings with a refreshing and vibrant fruit salad brimming with the sweetness of mangoes, peaches, and crisp apple slices. This delightful combination not only tantalizes your taste buds but also aligns perfectly with a low histamine diet.

Ingredients:
- Mango
- Peaches
- Apple

Preparation Method:
Step 1 - Preparing Mango:
- Peel the mango and cut it into bite-sized cubes.

Step 2 - Preparing Peaches:
- Wash the peaches thoroughly, remove the pit, and slice them into wedges or cubes.

Step 3 - Preparing Apples:
- Wash the apple, remove the core, and slice it into thin, manageable slices.

Portion Sizes: Aim for a balanced portion with equal parts of mango, peaches, and apple slices, typically around 1 cup each for a satisfying breakfast serving.

Storage and Handling Tips: Store any leftover fruit salad in an airtight container in the refrigerator for up to two days to maintain freshness. Keep fruits fresh by storing them in a cool, dry place or refrigerating them as necessary.

Substitutions: Feel free to include other low histamine fruits such as blueberries or apricots based on individual preferences and availability.

Hydration and Beverages: Accompany this fruit salad breakfast with water, herbal teas, or suitable fruit juices (avoiding citrus) to support hydration and enhance the morning refreshment.

Individual Tolerance: As individual tolerance levels can vary, monitor your body's response to different fruits. Adjust portion sizes or make fruit substitutions as needed to align with your specific dietary needs and prevent histamine reactions.

- Lunch: Turkey Lettuce Wraps & Roasted Beets Delight

Introduction: Dive into a light and satisfying lunch featuring turkey slices wrapped in crisp lettuce leaves, complemented by creamy cream cheese, alongside the earthy flavors of roasted beets. This combination offers a delightful low histamine meal to power you through the day.

Ingredients:
- Turkey slices (freshly cooked)
- Lettuce leaves
- Cream cheese (low histamine)
- Beets

Preparation Method:
Step 1 - Turkey Lettuce Wraps:
- Lay out the lettuce leaves.
- Spread a thin layer of cream cheese on each lettuce leaf.
- Place turkey slices on the lettuce leaves and roll them up into wraps.

Step 2 - Roasted Beets:
- Preheat the oven to 400°F (200°C).
- Wash and peel the beets, then cut them into cubes or wedges.
- Toss the beet pieces in a little oil and season with salt and pepper.
- Place the seasoned beets on a baking sheet and roast for about 25-30 minutes until tender and slightly caramelized.

Portion Sizes: Aim for 2-3 turkey lettuce wraps per serving, accompanied by a portion of roasted beets, about half to one cup, for a balanced and fulfilling lunch.

Storage and Handling Tips: Store any leftover turkey wraps and roasted beets in separate airtight containers in the refrigerator for up to 2-3 days. Ensure proper storage to maintain freshness.

Substitutions: For vegetarian or vegan options, replace turkey with tofu or tempeh slices marinated in low histamine sauces. Consider using dairy-free cream cheese alternatives if needed.

Hydration and Beverages: Pair this light lunch with water, herbal teas, or suitable fruit juices (avoiding citrus) to enhance hydration and complement the flavors.

Individual Tolerance: Monitor your body's response to turkey, cream cheese, and beets. Adjust portion sizes or consider alternative ingredients if needed to accommodate specific dietary needs and prevent histamine reactions.

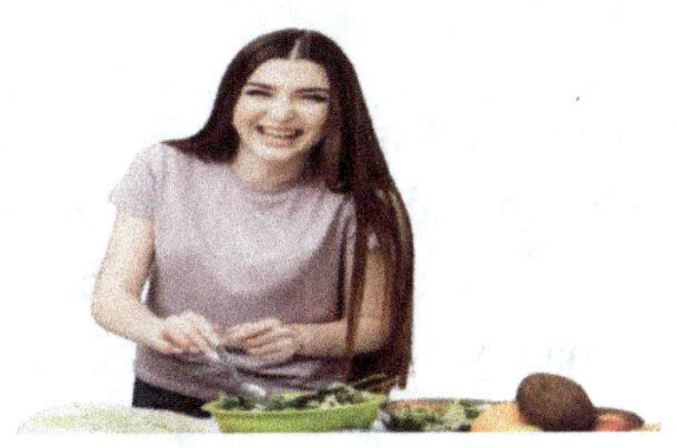

- Dinner: Grilled Chicken and Asparagus Delight with Cucumber Salad

Introduction: Embrace a delightful dinner featuring succulent grilled chicken, tender steamed asparagus, and a refreshing side salad of crisp cucumbers. This well-balanced meal caters to a low histamine diet while offering a delightful combination of flavors and textures.

Ingredients:
- Chicken breast (freshly cooked)
- Asparagus
- Cucumbers
- Salad greens (optional)
- Dressing (low histamine options)

Preparation Method:
Step 1 - Grilled Chicken:
- Preheat the grill to medium-high heat.
- Season the chicken breast with preferred low histamine herbs, salt, and pepper.
- Grill the chicken for about 6-8 minutes per side or until thoroughly cooked.

Step 2 - Steamed Asparagus:
- Trim the tough ends of the asparagus spears.
- Steam the asparagus in a steamer basket over boiling water for approximately 3-5 minutes until tender yet firm.

Step 3 - Cucumber Salad:
- Thinly slice the cucumbers.
- If desired, arrange the cucumber slices on a bed of salad greens.
- Drizzle with a low histamine dressing or a simple vinaigrette.

Portion Sizes: Aim for a palm-sized portion of grilled chicken, around 5-6 asparagus spears, and a serving of cucumber salad that suits your preference for a balanced dinner.

Storage and Handling Tips: Store any leftover grilled chicken, asparagus, and cucumber salad components separately in airtight containers in the refrigerator for up to 2-3 days.

Substitutions: Substitute chicken with grilled tofu, tempeh, or a low histamine fish for alternative protein options. Utilize a low histamine dressing or opt for a simple olive oil and vinegar dressing for the salad.

Hydration and Beverages: Complement this dinner with water, herbal teas, or suitable fruit juices (avoiding citrus) to complement the flavors and ensure proper hydration.

Individual Tolerance: Monitor your body's response to chicken, asparagus, cucumbers, and any dressings used. Adjust ingredients or portion sizes as needed to align with specific dietary needs and prevent histamine reactions.

Day 4

- Breakfast: Creamy Oatmeal Delight with Apricots

Introduction: Start your day with a cozy and satisfying breakfast featuring creamy oatmeal adorned with delightful sliced apricots and a dollop of creamy cream cheese. This flavorful combination offers a comforting and histamine-friendly morning meal.

Ingredients:
- Oats (low histamine)
- Apricots
- Cream cheese (low histamine)

Preparation Method:
Step 1 - Oatmeal:
- Prepare the oatmeal according to package instructions, using your preferred low histamine oats. Cook them in water or a low histamine milk substitute for added creaminess.

Step 2 - Sliced Apricots:
- Wash and slice the apricots into thin wedges or bite-sized pieces.

Step 3 - Cream Cheese Dollop:
- Once the oatmeal is cooked, serve it in a bowl.
- Top the oatmeal with sliced apricots and add a dollop of cream cheese.

Portion Sizes: Aim for a serving of oatmeal that aligns with your appetite, adding a suitable portion of sliced apricots and a modest dollop of cream cheese for flavor enhancement.

Storage and Handling Tips: Store any leftover sliced apricots and cream cheese in separate airtight containers in the refrigerator. Consume within a few days for optimal freshness.

Substitutions: For dairy-free or vegan alternatives, opt for dairy-free cream cheese options available in the market.

Hydration and Beverages: Enjoy this breakfast with water, herbal teas, or suitable fruit juices (avoiding citrus) to kickstart your day with adequate hydration.

Individual Tolerance: Monitor your body's response to apricots and cream cheese. Adjust portion sizes or consider alternative toppings if needed to accommodate specific dietary needs and prevent histamine reactions.

- Lunch: Wholesome Baked Fish & Sweet Potato Harmony with Steamed Broccoli

Introduction: Dive into a lunchtime feast that harmonizes the delightful flavors of baked fish with the comforting sweetness of roasted sweet potatoes, alongside the nourishing freshness of steamed broccoli. This balanced meal caters to a low histamine diet while offering a delightful blend of textures and tastes.

Ingredients:
- Fish filets (fresh or frozen)
- Sweet potatoes
- Broccoli

Preparation Method:
Step 1 - Baked Fish:
- Preheat the oven to 375°F (190°C).
- Season the fish filets with preferred low histamine herbs, salt, and pepper.
- Place the seasoned fish on a baking sheet lined with parchment paper.
- Bake for approximately 12-15 minutes until the fish flakes easily with a fork.

Step 2 - Roasted Sweet Potatoes:
- Wash and peel the sweet potatoes, then cut them into cubes or wedges.

- Toss the sweet potato pieces in a little oil and season with salt and preferred low histamine herbs.
- Place them on a baking sheet and roast in the oven at 400°F (200°C) for about 20-25 minutes until tender and caramelized.

Step 3 - Steamed Broccoli:
- Cut the broccoli into florets.
- Steam the broccoli in a steamer basket over boiling water for about 3-5 minutes until it's vibrant green and tender-crisp.

Portion Sizes: Aim for a palm-sized portion of fish, around one cup of roasted sweet potatoes, and a serving of steamed broccoli that suits your preference for a well-balanced lunch.

Storage and Handling Tips: Store any leftover baked fish, roasted sweet potatoes, and steamed broccoli in separate airtight containers in the refrigerator for up to 2-3 days.

Substitutions: Replace fish with another low histamine seafood option or tofu for alternative protein choices. Utilize olive oil or alternative low histamine oils for roasting sweet potatoes.

Hydration and Beverages: Accompany this lunch with water, herbal teas, or suitable fruit juices (avoiding citrus) to complement the meal and ensure proper hydration.

Individual Tolerance: Monitor your body's response to fish, sweet potatoes, and broccoli. Adjust ingredients or portion sizes as needed to accommodate specific dietary needs and prevent histamine reactions.

- Dinner: Herb-Infused Stir-Fried Vegetable Medley with Rice

Introduction: Immerse yourself in a delightful dinner experience with a vibrant stir-fried vegetable medley boasting the flavors of onions, squash, and asparagus, paired harmoniously with aromatic rice and fresh herbs of your choice. This dish celebrates the essence of low histamine ingredients while offering a burst of savory goodness.

Ingredients:
- Onions
- Squash
- Asparagus
- Rice (low histamine grain)
- Fresh herbs (of your choice)

Preparation Method:
Step 1 - Rice Preparation:
- Cook the rice according to package instructions using your preferred low histamine grain. Set aside once done.

Step 2 - Stir-Fried Vegetables:
- Chop the onions, squash, and asparagus into uniform sizes for even cooking.
- Heat a skillet or wok over medium-high heat with a small amount of oil.
- Add the onions, squash, and asparagus to the heated pan, stirring frequently for about 5-7 minutes until they are tender yet still crisp.

Step 3 - Herb Infusion:
- Finely chop or tear the fresh herbs of your choice.
- Once the vegetables are cooked, sprinkle the fresh herbs over the stir-fried medley and gently toss to infuse the flavors.

Portion Sizes: Aim for a balanced plate with around 1 cup of cooked rice and a generous serving of the stir-fried vegetable medley, adjusting according to your appetite.

Storage and Handling Tips: Store any leftover rice and stir-fried vegetables separately in airtight containers in the refrigerator for up to 2-3 days.

Substitutions: Feel free to add tofu, tempeh, or a low histamine protein of your choice to the stir-fried vegetables. Utilize low histamine sauces or seasonings for added flavor if preferred.

Hydration and Beverages: Pair this dinner with water, herbal teas, or suitable fruit juices (avoiding citrus) to complement the meal and maintain proper hydration.

Individual Tolerance: Monitor your body's response to the vegetables, rice, and herbs. Adjust ingredients or portion sizes as needed to accommodate specific dietary needs and prevent histamine reactions.

Day 5

- Breakfast: Scrumptious Yolk-Only Scrambled Eggs with Sautéed Onions and Sweet Potatoes

Introduction: Start your day with a satisfying breakfast featuring indulgent yolk-only scrambled eggs accompanied by the rich flavors of sautéed onions and the comforting sweetness of sweet potatoes. This delightful combination embraces low histamine foods to kickstart your morning with a hearty meal.

Ingredients:
- Eggs (using yolks only)
- Onions
- Sweet potatoes

Preparation Method:
Step 1 - Yolk-Only Scrambled Eggs:
- Crack the eggs and separate the yolks from the whites.

- Whisk the egg yolks gently in a bowl.
- Heat a non-stick skillet over medium heat, add a touch of oil if needed, and pour in the whisked yolks.
- Stir continuously until the eggs are softly scrambled and cooked to your desired consistency.

Step 2 - Sautéed Onions and Sweet Potatoes:
- Peel and dice the sweet potatoes into small cubes.
- Heat a skillet with a small amount of oil over medium heat.
- Add diced onions and sweet potatoes to the skillet.
- Sauté the mixture, stirring occasionally, until the sweet potatoes are tender and lightly browned, usually around 10-12 minutes.

Portion Sizes: Aim for a serving size of 2-3 egg yolks scrambled, along with a portion of sautéed onions and sweet potatoes that suits your breakfast appetite.

Storage and Handling Tips: Store any leftover sautéed onions and sweet potatoes in an airtight container in the refrigerator for up to 2-3 days.

Substitutions: For a vegan option, consider using tofu or tempeh instead of eggs. Replace sweet potatoes with other low histamine vegetables like squash or asparagus.

Hydration and Beverages: Pair this breakfast with water, herbal teas, or suitable fruit juices (avoiding citrus) for a refreshing start to your day.

Individual Tolerance: Monitor your body's response to eggs, onions, and sweet potatoes. Adjust ingredients or portion sizes as needed to accommodate specific dietary needs and prevent histamine reactions.

- Lunch: Turkey Slices Paired with a Refreshing Cucumber and Beet Salad

Introduction: Elevate your lunchtime with the lean protein goodness of turkey slices, paired alongside a refreshing side salad boasting the crispness of cucumbers and the earthy richness of beets. This low histamine meal offers a delightful blend of flavors and textures for a satisfying lunch.

Ingredients:
- Turkey slices (freshly cooked)
- Cucumbers
- Beets

Preparation Method:
Step 1 - Turkey Slices:
- Use freshly cooked turkey slices. If required, warm them briefly in a skillet or microwave.

Step 2 - Cucumber and Beet Salad:
- Wash and peel the cucumbers and beets.
- Thinly slice the cucumbers and cut the beets into bite-sized pieces or slices.

- Arrange the cucumber slices and beet pieces in a serving bowl.

Portion Sizes: Aim for a balanced lunch with a serving size of turkey slices that meets your protein needs, alongside a satisfying portion of cucumber and beet salad.

Storage and Handling Tips: Store any leftover turkey slices and salad components separately in airtight containers in the refrigerator for up to 2-3 days.

Substitutions: For vegetarian or vegan options, consider using plant-based protein alternatives or roasted tofu slices in place of turkey. Opt for a dairy-free dressing if desired.

Hydration and Beverages: Accompany this lunch with water, herbal teas, or suitable fruit juices (avoiding citrus) to complement the meal and maintain hydration levels.

Individual Tolerance: Monitor your body's response to turkey, cucumbers, and beets. Adjust portion sizes or consider alternative ingredients if needed to accommodate specific dietary needs and prevent histamine reactions.

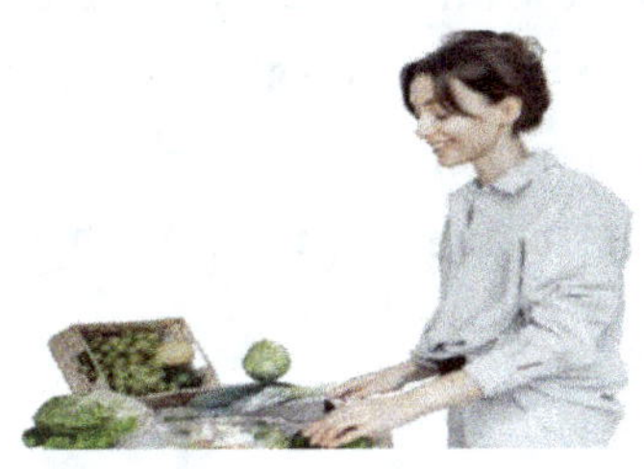

- Dinner: Grilled Chicken Harmony with Mashed Potatoes and Sautéed Asparagus

Introduction: Indulge in a delightful dinner featuring succulent grilled chicken complemented by comforting mashed potatoes and vibrant sautéed asparagus. This balanced meal brings together the flavors of low histamine ingredients for a satisfying dining experience.

Ingredients:
- Chicken breast (freshly grilled)
- Potatoes
- Asparagus

Preparation Method:
Step 1 - Grilled Chicken:
- Preheat the grill to medium-high heat.
- Season the chicken breast with preferred low histamine herbs, salt, and pepper.
- Grill the chicken for about 6-8 minutes per side or until thoroughly cooked.

Step 2 - Mashed Potatoes:
- Peel and chop the potatoes into evenly sized chunks.
- Boil the potato chunks in a pot of salted water until tender, usually around 15-20 minutes.
- Drain the potatoes, mash them using a masher or fork, and season to taste.

Step 3 - Sautéed Asparagus:
- Trim the tough ends of the asparagus spears.
- Heat a skillet with a small amount of oil over medium heat.
- Add the asparagus spears to the skillet and sauté for 5-7 minutes until they are tender-crisp.

Portion Sizes: Aim for a palm-sized portion of grilled chicken, a serving of mashed potatoes equivalent to one medium-sized potato, and a generous portion of sautéed asparagus for a balanced dinner.

Storage and Handling Tips: Store any leftover grilled chicken, mashed potatoes, and asparagus separately in airtight containers in the refrigerator for up to 2-3 days.

Substitutions: Replace chicken with grilled tofu, tempeh, or a low histamine fish for alternative protein options. Utilize olive oil or alternative low histamine oils for sautéing asparagus.

Hydration and Beverages: Pair this dinner with water, herbal teas, or suitable fruit juices (avoiding citrus) to complement the meal and maintain proper hydration.

Individual Tolerance: Monitor your body's response to chicken, potatoes, and asparagus. Adjust ingredients or portion sizes as needed to accommodate specific dietary needs and prevent histamine reactions.

Day 6

- Breakfast: Blueberry-Mango-Apple Smoothie: A Refreshing Morning Treat

Introduction: Start your day on a vibrant note with a luscious fruit smoothie brimming with the goodness of blueberries, mango, and apple. This invigorating blend offers a burst of flavors and essential nutrients, ideal for a low histamine breakfast.

Ingredients:
- Blueberries
- Mango
- Apple

Preparation Method:
Step 1 - Fruit Preparation:
- Wash and prepare the fruits.
- Peel and dice the mango and apple into manageable chunks.

Step 2 - Smoothie Creation:
- In a blender, combine the prepared blueberries, diced mango, and apple chunks.
- Blend until smooth and creamy, adjusting the consistency with water if desired.

Portion Sizes: Aim for a serving size that suits your appetite, ensuring a balanced intake of the fruit smoothie for breakfast.

Storage and Handling Tips: Consume the fruit smoothie immediately for freshness and optimal taste. If any leftover, store it in an airtight container in the refrigerator for a few hours. Shake or stir before consuming.

Substitutions: Consider adding a splash of pasteurized milk or a dairy-free alternative for a creamier texture. You can also incorporate a low histamine protein powder or seeds for added nutrition.

Hydration and Beverages: Accompany this smoothie with water, herbal teas, or suitable fruit juices (avoiding citrus) for a hydrating start to your day.

Individual Tolerance: Monitor your body's response to blueberries, mangoes, and apples. Adjust ingredients or portion sizes as needed to accommodate specific dietary needs and prevent histamine reactions.

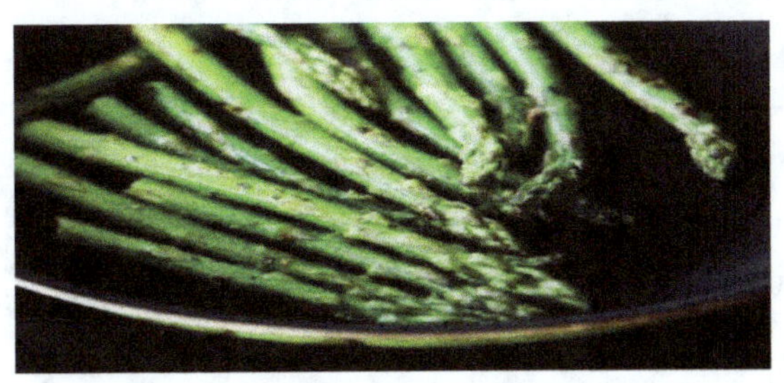

- Lunch: Baked Fish Harmony with Steamed Broccoli and Roasted Sweet Potatoes

Introduction: Enjoy a delightful lunch featuring tender baked fish alongside the vibrant goodness of steamed broccoli and the comforting sweetness of roasted sweet potatoes. This low histamine meal brings together a blend of flavors and nutrients for a satisfying midday meal.

Ingredients:
- Fish filets (fresh or frozen)
- Broccoli
- Sweet potatoes

Preparation Method:
Step 1 - Baked Fish:
- Preheat the oven to 375°F (190°C).
- Season the fish filets with preferred low histamine herbs, salt, and pepper.
- Place the seasoned fish on a baking sheet lined with parchment paper.
- Bake for approximately 12-15 minutes until the fish is cooked through and flakes easily with a fork.

Step 2 - Steamed Broccoli:
- Wash and cut the broccoli into florets.
- Steam the broccoli in a steamer basket over boiling water for about 5-7 minutes until it's tender yet crisp.

Step 3 - Roasted Sweet Potatoes:
- Peel and dice the sweet potatoes into bite-sized cubes.
- Toss the sweet potato cubes with a small amount of oil, salt, and preferred low histamine herbs.
- Roast in the oven at 400°F (200°C) for 20-25 minutes or until they are tender and golden.

Portion Sizes: Aim for a portion of baked fish that satisfies your appetite, along with a generous serving of steamed broccoli and a suitable portion of roasted sweet potatoes for a balanced lunch.

Storage and Handling Tips: Store any leftover baked fish, steamed broccoli, and roasted sweet potatoes separately in airtight containers in the refrigerator for up to 2-3 days.

Substitutions: Consider using a different low histamine vegetable in place of broccoli or opt for other low histamine root vegetables instead of sweet potatoes.

Hydration and Beverages: Complement this lunch with water, herbal teas, or suitable fruit juices (avoiding citrus) to balance the meal and maintain proper hydration.

Individual Tolerance: Monitor your body's response to fish, broccoli, and sweet potatoes. Adjust ingredients or portion sizes as needed to accommodate specific dietary needs and prevent histamine reactions.

- Dinner: Flavorful Turkey Stir-Fry Infused with Squash, Onions, and Herbs over Rice

Introduction: Indulge in a delightful dinner featuring a fragrant and savory turkey stir-fry enriched with squash, onions, and aromatic herbs served atop a bed of rice. This low histamine meal offers a delightful blend of textures and flavors for a satisfying dining experience.

Ingredients:
- Turkey slices (freshly cooked)
- Squash
- Onions
- Herbs (such as parsley, thyme, or basil)
- Rice (of your choice)

Preparation Method:
Step 1 - Turkey Stir-Fry:
- Slice the cooked turkey into thin strips or bite-sized pieces.
- Heat a skillet or wok over medium-high heat and add a small amount of oil.
- Add the turkey slices to the skillet and stir-fry until they are lightly browned and cooked through.
- Remove the turkey from the skillet and set it aside.

Step 2 - Vegetable Stir-Fry:
- Peel and dice the squash and onions into even pieces.
- In the same skillet, add a bit more oil if needed and sauté the diced squash and onions until they are tender yet crisp.

- Once the vegetables are almost done, return the cooked turkey to the skillet.

Step 3 - Herb Infusion and Rice Preparation:
- Add the herbs to the turkey and vegetable mixture, allowing them to infuse their flavors for a minute or two.
- Prepare the rice according to package instructions to serve as the base for the stir-fry.

Portion Sizes: Aim for a balanced portion of turkey stir-fry served over a suitable serving of rice to create a fulfilling dinner.

Storage and Handling Tips: Store any leftover turkey stir-fry and rice separately in airtight containers in the refrigerator for up to 2-3 days.

Substitutions: Explore using alternative low histamine vegetables like asparagus or bell peppers in place of squash or consider brown rice or quinoa as a substitute for rice.

Hydration and Beverages: Complement this dinner with water, herbal teas, or suitable fruit juices (avoiding citrus) to accompany the meal and maintain proper hydration.

Individual Tolerance: Monitor your body's response to turkey, squash, onions, and herbs. Adjust ingredients or portion sizes as needed to accommodate specific dietary needs and prevent histamine reactions.

Day 7

- Breakfast: Peaches & Cream Oatmeal Elegance for Breakfast

Introduction: Embrace a delightful morning with a bowl of comforting oatmeal adorned with the sweet, juicy allure of sliced peaches and a touch of creamy pasteurized milk. This breakfast combines the wholesomeness of oats with the succulence of peaches, perfect for a low histamine start to your day.

Ingredients:
- Oats (low histamine)
- Peaches
- Pasteurized milk

Preparation Method:
Step 1 - Oatmeal Preparation:
- Cook the oatmeal according to package instructions, using your preferred low histamine oats. Use water or pasteurized milk for added creaminess.

Step 2 - Sliced Peaches:
- Wash the peaches thoroughly and slice them into thin wedges or bite-sized pieces.

Step 3 - Peaches & Cream Assembly:
- Once the oatmeal is cooked, serve it in a bowl.
- Top the oatmeal with the freshly sliced peaches.
- Add a splash of pasteurized milk for a creamy finish.

Portion Sizes: Aim for a serving of oatmeal that satisfies your appetite, along with a suitable portion of sliced peaches and a modest splash of pasteurized milk to enhance the flavors.

Storage and Handling Tips: Store any leftover sliced peaches in an airtight container in the refrigerator for a day or two. Ensure the oatmeal is stored in a sealed container and consumed within 2-3 days.

Substitutions: For dairy-free or vegan options, consider using almond milk, oat milk, or coconut milk as alternatives to pasteurized milk.

Hydration and Beverages: Enjoy this breakfast with water, herbal teas, or suitable fruit juices (avoiding citrus) to complement the flavors and ensure proper hydration.

Individual Tolerance: Monitor your body's response to peaches and pasteurized milk. Adjust ingredients or portion sizes as needed to accommodate specific dietary needs and prevent histamine reactions.

- Lunch: Creamy Grilled Chicken Salad Infused with Cucumber and Beets

Introduction: Delight in a satisfying lunch experience featuring tender grilled chicken atop a vibrant salad bed adorned with crisp cucumbers and earthy beets. Elevate the flavors with a creamy dressing crafted from the richness of cream cheese, offering a delightful ensemble of textures and tastes for a low histamine meal.

Ingredients:
- Grilled chicken (sliced or shredded)
- Cucumbers
- Beets
- Cream cheese (for the dressing)

Preparation Method:
Step 1 - Grilled Chicken:
- Grill the chicken breasts until they are fully cooked. Let them cool before slicing or shredding for the salad.

Step 2 - Salad Assembly:
- Wash and slice the cucumbers into thin rounds.
- Peel and cut the beets into bite-sized pieces or slices.
- Arrange a bed of salad greens and top it with sliced or shredded grilled chicken, cucumber slices, and beet pieces.

Step 3 - Creamy Dressing:
- In a bowl, blend the cream cheese until smooth and creamy.
- Add a touch of water or preferred low histamine liquid to achieve the desired dressing consistency.
- Drizzle the creamy dressing over the salad just before serving.

Portion Sizes: Aim for a satisfying portion of salad greens topped with a generous serving of grilled chicken, cucumber slices, beets, and a modest amount of creamy dressing.

Storage and Handling Tips: Store any leftover salad components and dressing separately in airtight containers in the refrigerator. Consume within 1-2 days for optimal freshness.

Substitutions: For a dairy-free or vegan alternative, consider using a dairy-free creamy substitute or avocado-based dressing for the salad.

Hydration and Beverages: Complement this salad with water, herbal teas, or suitable fruit juices (avoiding citrus) to balance the meal and ensure proper hydration.

Individual Tolerance: Monitor your body's response to chicken, cucumbers, beets, and cream cheese. Adjust ingredients or portion sizes as needed to accommodate specific dietary needs and prevent histamine reactions.

- Dinner: Baked Salmon Harmony with Creamy Mashed Potatoes and Steamed Asparagus

Introduction: Treat yourself to a delectable dinner featuring succulent baked salmon paired with velvety mashed potatoes and tender steamed asparagus. This low histamine meal boasts a combination of flavors and textures for a delightful dining experience.

Ingredients:
- Salmon filets (fresh or frozen)
- Potatoes
- Asparagus

Preparation Method:
Step 1 - Baked Salmon:
- Preheat the oven to 375°F (190°C).
- Season the salmon filets with preferred low histamine herbs, salt, and pepper.
- Place the seasoned salmon on a baking sheet lined with parchment paper.
- Bake for approximately 12-15 minutes until the salmon flakes easily with a fork.

Step 2 - Creamy Mashed Potatoes:
- Peel and chop the potatoes into evenly sized chunks.
- Boil the potato chunks in a pot of salted water until tender, usually around 15-20 minutes.

- Drain the potatoes, mash them using a masher or fork, and season to taste.

Step 3 - Steamed Asparagus:
- Trim the tough ends of the asparagus spears.
- Steam the asparagus in a steamer basket over boiling water for about 3-5 minutes until they are tender-crisp.

Portion Sizes: Aim for a palm-sized portion of baked salmon, a serving of mashed potatoes equivalent to one medium-sized potato, and a satisfying portion of steamed asparagus for a balanced dinner.

Storage and Handling Tips: Store any leftover baked salmon, mashed potatoes, and steamed asparagus separately in airtight containers in the refrigerator for up to 2-3 days.

Substitutions: Replace salmon with another low histamine seafood option or grilled tofu for alternative protein choices. Utilize olive oil or alternative low histamine oils for seasoning.

Hydration and Beverages: Accompany this dinner with water, herbal teas, or suitable fruit juices (avoiding citrus) to complement the meal and maintain proper hydration.

Individual Tolerance: Monitor your body's response to salmon, potatoes, and asparagus. Adjust ingredients or portion sizes as needed to accommodate specific dietary needs and prevent histamine reactions.

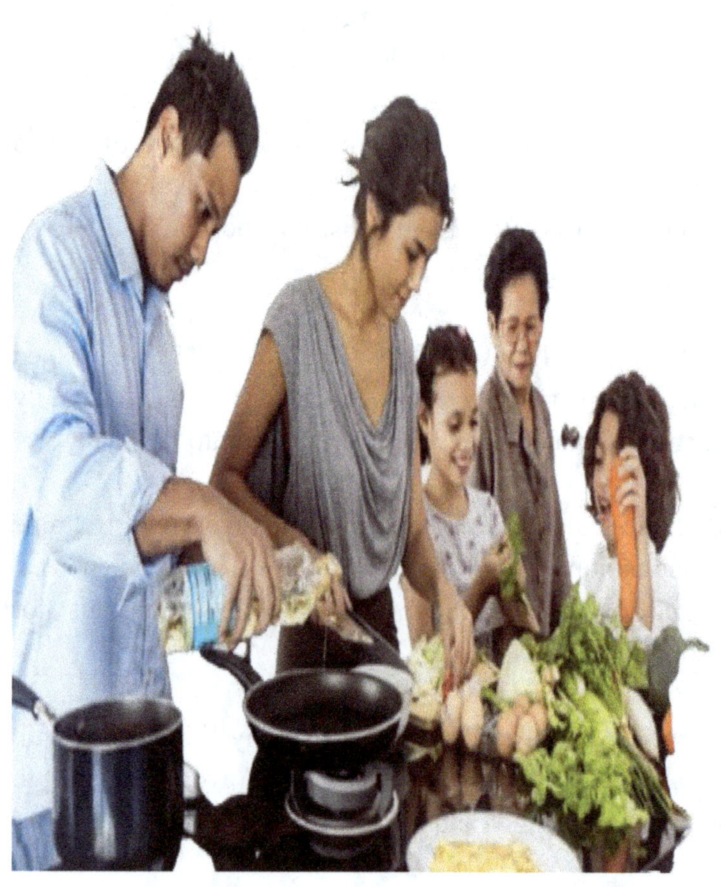

WEEK 2

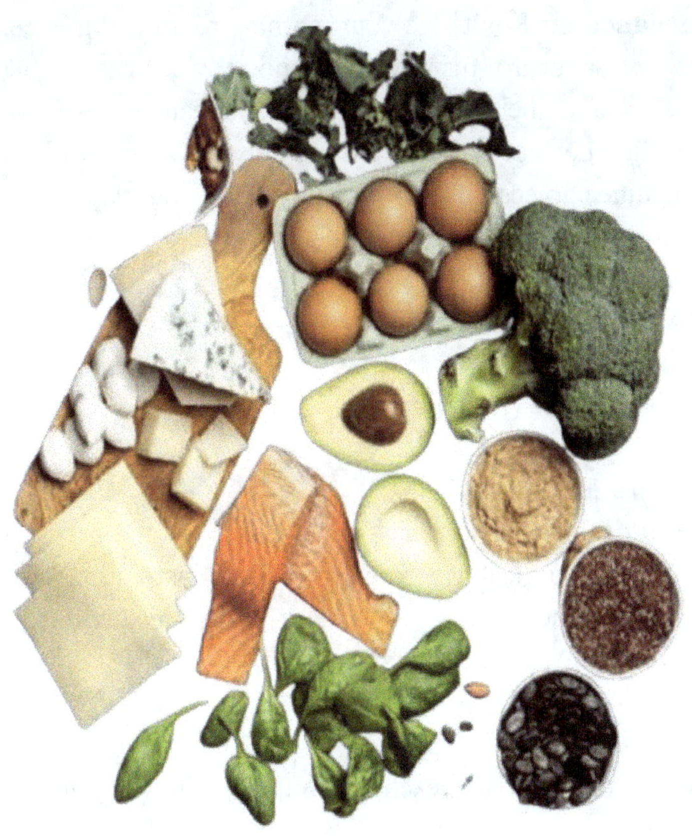

Day 8

- Breakfast: Peaches & Cream Oatmeal Bliss for Breakfast

Introduction: Revitalize your morning routine with a cozy bowl of oatmeal infused with the juicy sweetness of sliced peaches and the creamy richness of cream cheese. This breakfast not only offers comfort but also aligns with low histamine choices for a nourishing start to your day.

Ingredients:
- Oats (low histamine)
- Peaches
- Cream cheese (for topping)

Preparation Method:
Step 1 - Oatmeal Preparation:
- Cook the oatmeal according to package instructions using low histamine oats. Use water or a low histamine milk alternative for added creaminess.

Step 2 - Sliced Peaches:
- Wash and slice the peaches into thin wedges or bite-sized pieces.

Step 3 - Peaches & Cream Topping:
- Once the oatmeal is cooked, serve it in a bowl.
- Top the oatmeal with the freshly sliced peaches.

- Add a dollop of cream cheese on top for a delightful creamy touch.

Portion Sizes: Opt for a serving of oatmeal that satisfies your appetite, coupled with an adequate portion of sliced peaches and a modest dollop of cream cheese for a balanced breakfast.

Storage and Handling Tips: Use fresh peaches and consume the oatmeal immediately for optimal taste. Store any leftover oatmeal in an airtight container and consume within 1-2 days.

Substitutions: For dairy-free or vegan options, consider using a dairy-free cream cheese substitute or coconut cream for a creamy topping.

Hydration and Beverages: Accompany this breakfast with water, herbal teas, or suitable fruit juices (avoiding citrus) to complement the flavors and maintain proper hydration.

Individual Tolerance: Monitor your body's response to peaches and cream cheese. Adjust ingredients or portion sizes as needed to accommodate specific dietary needs and prevent histamine reactions.

- Lunch: Grilled Turkey Slices with Crisp Salad and Animal Fat Herb Vinaigrette

Introduction: Elevate your lunch hour with the succulent taste of grilled turkey slices served alongside a refreshing salad featuring crisp cucumbers and zesty onions. Enhance the flavors with a tantalizing vinaigrette crafted from animal fats and aromatic herbs, all aligned with low histamine choices for a satisfying midday meal.

Ingredients:
- Turkey slices (grilled)
- Cucumbers
- Onions
- Animal fats (for vinaigrette)
- Herbs (such as parsley, thyme, or basil)

Preparation Method:
Step 1 - Grilled Turkey Slices:
- Grill the turkey slices until they are cooked through and possess a golden brown exterior. Let them cool before slicing.

Step 2 - Salad Assembly:
- Wash and slice the cucumbers into thin rounds.
- Peel and slice the onions into thin strips or rings.

Step 3 - Animal Fat Herb Vinaigrette:
- In a bowl, combine the animal fats with finely chopped herbs to create the vinaigrette.
- Whisk the mixture until it forms a smooth and well-blended dressing.

Step 4 - Salad Plating:
- Arrange the grilled turkey slices on a plate.
- Surround them with the cucumber slices and onion strips.
- Drizzle the herb-infused animal fat vinaigrette over the salad just before serving.

Portion Sizes: Opt for a portion of grilled turkey slices that satiates your hunger, alongside a generous serving of cucumber and onion salad. Use a suitable amount of vinaigrette to complement the flavors.

Storage and Handling Tips: Consume the salad immediately after adding the vinaigrette for optimal taste. Store any leftover components separately and consume within 1-2 days.

Substitutions: Explore using a different low histamine protein source instead of turkey or switch to a different low histamine dressing option based on individual preferences or dietary needs.

Hydration and Beverages: Pair this lunch with water, herbal teas, or suitable fruit juices (avoiding citrus) for a refreshing accompaniment to the meal.

Individual Tolerance: Monitor your body's response to turkey, cucumbers, onions, and animal fats. Adjust ingredients or portion sizes as needed to accommodate specific dietary needs and prevent histamine reactions.

- Dinner: Baked Cod Delight with Sautéed Squash and Steamed Asparagus

Introduction: Treat yourself to a delightful dinner featuring tender baked cod paired with the subtle flavors of sautéed squash and the freshness of steamed asparagus. This low histamine meal provides a wholesome and flavorsome dining experience.

Ingredients:
- Cod filets (fresh or frozen)
- Squash
- Asparagus

Preparation Method:
Step 1 - Baked Cod:
- Preheat the oven to 375°F (190°C).
- Season the cod filets with preferred low histamine herbs, salt, and pepper.

- Place the seasoned cod on a baking sheet lined with parchment paper.
- Bake for approximately 12-15 minutes or until the cod is flaky and thoroughly cooked.

Step 2 - Sautéed Squash:
- Wash and dice the squash into uniform pieces.
- Heat a pan over medium heat, add a small amount of oil, and sauté the diced squash until it's tender yet retains a slight crunch. Season as desired.

Step 3 - Steamed Asparagus:
- Trim the tough ends of the asparagus spears.
- Steam the asparagus in a steamer basket over boiling water for about 3-5 minutes until they are tender-crisp.

Portion Sizes: Opt for a portion of baked cod that suits your appetite, coupled with a generous serving of sautéed squash and an appropriate portion of steamed asparagus for a balanced dinner.

Storage and Handling Tips: Store any leftover baked cod, sautéed squash, and steamed asparagus separately in airtight containers in the refrigerator for up to 2-3 days.

Substitutions: Swap cod with another low histamine fish or seafood option if desired. Consider using alternative low histamine vegetables to replace squash or asparagus based on personal preferences or availability.

Hydration and Beverages: Accompany this dinner with water, herbal teas, or suitable fruit juices (avoiding citrus) to complement the meal and maintain proper hydration.

Individual Tolerance: Monitor your body's response to cod, squash, and asparagus. Adjust ingredients or portion sizes as needed to accommodate specific dietary needs and prevent histamine reactions.

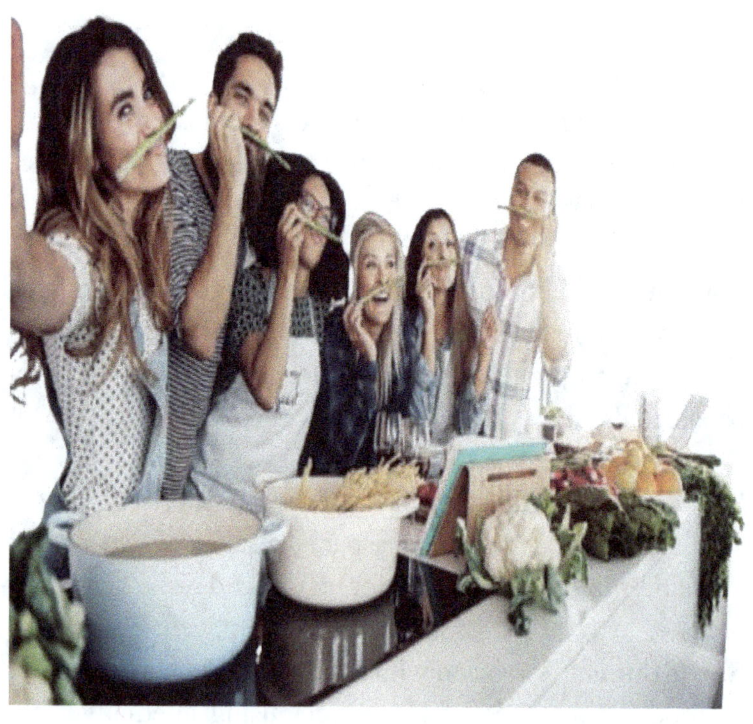

Day 9

- Breakfast: Yolk-licious Scrambled Eggs with Sautéed Onions and a Mango Sidekick

Introduction: Start your day with a savory breakfast featuring sumptuous scrambled eggs, prepared using yolks for a low histamine twist, accompanied by the aromatic allure of sautéed onions. Pair this with the sweet and juicy freshness of sliced mango for a delightful morning meal.

Ingredients:
- Eggs (yolks only)
- Onions
- Mango

Preparation Method:
Step 1 - Scrambled Eggs:
- Separate the egg yolks from the whites.
- Whisk the egg yolks in a bowl until smooth.
- Cook the yolks in a pan over low heat, stirring gently until they reach the desired consistency for scrambled eggs.

Step 2 - Sautéed Onions:
- Peel and chop the onions finely.
- Heat a pan with a small amount of oil or butter over medium heat.
- Sauté the chopped onions until they turn golden brown and slightly caramelized.

Step 3 - Sliced Mango Side:
- Wash and peel the mango. Slice it into desirable pieces.

Portion Sizes: Aim for a balanced portion of scrambled egg yolks with sautéed onions, complemented by an appropriate serving of sliced mango to create a fulfilling breakfast.

Storage and Handling Tips: Consume the meal immediately for optimal taste. Store any leftovers separately in airtight containers in the refrigerator for up to a day.

Substitutions: For those seeking a vegan or vegetarian option, consider using tofu or a plant-based egg substitute in place of eggs. Substitute the mango with other low histamine fruits like peaches or apricots if preferred.

Hydration and Beverages: Accompany this breakfast with water, herbal teas, or suitable fruit juices (avoiding citrus) to complement the flavors and maintain proper hydration.

Individual Tolerance: Monitor your body's response to egg yolks, onions, and mango. Adjust ingredients or portion sizes as needed to accommodate specific dietary needs and prevent histamine reactions.

- Lunch: Grilled Chicken Salad Enhanced with Roasted Beets and Creamy Herb Dressing

Introduction: Elevate your lunch experience with a flavorful grilled chicken salad harmonized by the earthy sweetness of roasted beets and adorned with a luscious creamy dressing infused with cream cheese and fragrant herbs. This low histamine salad offers a delightful blend of textures and flavors for a satisfying midday meal.

Ingredients:
- Grilled chicken (freshly cooked)
- Roasted beets
- Cream cheese (for dressing)
- Herbs (such as parsley, thyme, or basil)

Preparation Method:
Step 1 - Grilled Chicken Preparation:
- Grill the chicken until it's cooked thoroughly and has a delightful smoky flavor. Once cooked, let it cool before slicing it into strips or bite-sized pieces.

Step 2 - Roasted Beets:
- Preheat the oven to 400°F (200°C).
- Wash and peel the beets, then cut them into uniform pieces.
- Place the beet pieces on a baking sheet, drizzle with a small amount of oil, and roast them in the oven for approximately 20-30 minutes or until tender.

Step 3 - Creamy Herb Dressing:
- Mix the cream cheese with finely chopped herbs in a bowl to create the creamy dressing. Adjust the consistency with a little bit of water if needed.

Step 4 - Salad Assembly:
- Arrange the grilled chicken and roasted beets on a plate or in a salad bowl.
- Drizzle the creamy herb dressing generously over the salad just before serving.

Portion Sizes: Aim for a balanced portion of grilled chicken and roasted beets with an adequate serving of creamy herb dressing to dress the salad.

Storage and Handling Tips: Prepare the salad just before consuming for optimal taste. Store any leftover components separately in airtight containers in the refrigerator for up to 1-2 days.

Substitutions: For dairy-free or vegan preferences, opt for a dairy-free cream cheese alternative or a plant-based creamy dressing option. Explore using alternative low histamine vegetables to replace roasted beets according to personal preferences or availability.

Hydration and Beverages: Complement this salad with water, herbal teas, or suitable fruit juices (avoiding citrus) to accompany the meal and maintain proper hydration.

Individual Tolerance: Monitor your body's response to grilled chicken, roasted beets, cream cheese, and herbs. Adjust ingredients or portion sizes as needed to accommodate specific dietary needs and prevent histamine reactions.

- Dinner: Turkey Stir-Fry Infused with Broccoli, Onions, and Rice

Introduction: Delight your taste buds with a wholesome turkey stir-fry brimming with vibrant vegetables like broccoli and onions, served alongside a bed of comforting rice. This low histamine dinner offers a perfect blend of protein and vegetables for a satisfying and flavorful meal.

Ingredients:
- Turkey (sliced or diced)
- Broccoli
- Onions
- Rice

Preparation Method:
Step 1 - Turkey Prep:
- Slice or dice the turkey into bite-sized pieces for the stir-fry.

Step 2 - Stir-Fry Assembly:
- Heat a pan or wok over medium-high heat and add a small amount of oil.

- Stir-fry the turkey pieces until they are cooked through and lightly browned.
- Add in the broccoli florets and sliced onions to the pan, continuing to stir-fry until they are tender yet crisp.

Step 3 - Rice Preparation:
- Prepare the rice separately following package instructions or your preferred method.

Step 4 - Plating:
- Serve the flavorful turkey stir-fry alongside a portion of rice, creating a balanced and fulfilling meal.

Portion Sizes: Opt for a balanced serving of turkey stir-fry, ensuring a generous amount of vegetables and a suitable portion of rice for a satisfying dinner.

Storage and Handling Tips: Consume the stir-fry immediately for optimal taste. Store any leftovers separately in airtight containers in the refrigerator for up to 1-2 days.

Substitutions: Substitute turkey with other low histamine protein sources like chicken or tofu. Replace broccoli or onions with alternative low histamine vegetables based on personal preferences or availability.

Hydration and Beverages: Accompany this dinner with water, herbal teas, or suitable fruit juices (avoiding citrus) to complement the meal and maintain proper hydration.

Individual Tolerance: Monitor your body's response to turkey, broccoli, onions, and rice. Adjust ingredients or portion sizes as needed to accommodate specific dietary needs and prevent histamine reactions.

Day 10

- Breakfast: Fresh and Fruity Morning Delight: Blueberry-Apple Fruit Salad

Introduction: Brighten up your morning with a refreshing and nutritious fruit salad, combining the juiciness of blueberries and the crispness of apple slices. A delicate drizzle of pasteurized milk adds a creamy touch to this delightful breakfast.

Ingredients:
- Blueberries
- Apple slices
- Pasteurized milk

Preparation Method:
Step 1 - Fruit Preparation:
- Rinse the blueberries thoroughly and pat them dry.
- Core the apple and slice it into thin, bite-sized pieces.

Step 2 - Salad Assembly:
- Combine the fresh blueberries and apple slices in a bowl.

Step 3 - Drizzle with Milk:
- Add a subtle drizzle of pasteurized milk over the fruit salad for a creamy finish.

Portion Sizes: Create a balanced fruit salad by combining an appropriate quantity of blueberries and apple slices, complemented by a light drizzle of pasteurized milk.

Storage and Handling Tips: Assemble and consume the fruit salad immediately for optimal freshness. Store any leftover fruits in separate airtight containers in the refrigerator and add milk just before eating.

Substitutions: Swap pasteurized milk with a dairy-free alternative or yogurt for a creamy twist, catering to specific dietary preferences or lactose intolerance.

Hydration and Beverages: Pair this breakfast with water, herbal teas, or suitable fruit juices (avoiding citrus) to complement the fruit salad and maintain hydration levels.

Individual Tolerance: Monitor your body's response to blueberries, apple slices, and pasteurized milk. Adjust ingredients or portion sizes as needed to accommodate specific dietary needs and prevent histamine reactions.

- Lunch: Baked Fish Harmony with Mashed Sweet Potatoes and Steamed Broccoli

Introduction: Indulge in a harmonious lunch featuring baked fish paired with velvety mashed sweet potatoes and a nutritious side of steamed broccoli. This meal not only satisfies your taste buds but also offers a nutritious and comforting dining experience.

Ingredients:
- Fish (fresh or frozen)
- Sweet potatoes
- Broccoli

Preparation Method:
Step 1 - Baked Fish:
- Preheat the oven to 375°F (190°C).
- Season the fish filets with your preferred low histamine herbs and spices.
- Place the seasoned fish on a baking tray lined with parchment paper.
- Bake in the preheated oven for about 15-20 minutes or until the fish is cooked through and flakes easily with a fork.

Step 2 - Mashed Sweet Potatoes:
- Peel and dice the sweet potatoes into cubes.
- Boil the sweet potato cubes in a pot of water until they are tender.

- Drain the water and mash the sweet potatoes using a fork or potato masher. Season as desired.

Step 3 - Steamed Broccoli:
- Wash the broccoli and cut it into florets.
- Steam the broccoli in a steamer basket over boiling water for approximately 3-5 minutes or until it's tender yet retains some crunch.

Portion Sizes: Aim for a balanced plate with a suitable portion of baked fish, a serving of mashed sweet potatoes, and a side of steamed broccoli for a well-rounded lunch.

Storage and Handling Tips: Consume the meal immediately for optimal taste. Store any leftovers separately in airtight containers in the refrigerator for up to 1-2 days.

Substitutions: Swap sweet potatoes with regular potatoes or another low histamine vegetable if preferred. Consider using another type of low histamine fish based on availability and personal taste.

Hydration and Beverages: Accompany this lunch with water, herbal teas, or suitable fruit juices (avoiding citrus) to complement the meal and maintain proper hydration.

Individual Tolerance: Monitor your body's response to fish, sweet potatoes, and broccoli. Adjust ingredients or portion sizes as needed to accommodate specific dietary needs and prevent histamine reactions.

- Dinner: Grilled Chicken Perfection with Roasted Squash and Rice Harmony

Introduction: Enjoy a delectable dinner comprising succulent grilled chicken complemented by the rustic sweetness of roasted squash and a comforting side of rice. This satisfying meal is a delightful blend of flavors and textures for a fulfilling dining experience.

Ingredients:
- Chicken (preferably boneless)
- Squash
- Rice

Preparation Method:
Step 1 - Grilled Chicken:
- Season the chicken with your preferred low histamine herbs and spices.
- Grill the seasoned chicken over medium-high heat until it's thoroughly cooked, maintaining juiciness.

Step 2 - Roasted Squash:
- Preheat the oven to 400°F (200°C).
- Wash and slice the squash into desired shapes.

- Place the squash slices on a baking sheet, drizzle with a touch of oil, and roast in the oven for approximately 20-25 minutes or until tender and caramelized.

Step 3 - Rice Preparation:
- Cook the rice separately following package instructions or your preferred method.

Step 4 - Plating:
- Arrange the grilled chicken on the plate alongside a portion of roasted squash and a serving of rice for a balanced and wholesome dinner.

Portion Sizes: Strive for a well-proportioned plate with an adequate serving of grilled chicken, a portion of roasted squash, and an appropriate amount of rice to create a satiating dinner.

Storage and Handling Tips: Enjoy the meal immediately for optimal taste. Store any leftover components separately in airtight containers in the refrigerator for up to 1-2 days.

Substitutions: Consider swapping squash with another low histamine vegetable, such as asparagus or broccoli, to suit personal preferences or availability.

Hydration and Beverages: Pair this dinner with water, herbal teas, or suitable fruit juices (avoiding citrus) to complement the meal and maintain proper hydration.

Individual Tolerance: Monitor your body's response to chicken, squash, and rice. Adjust ingredients or portion sizes as needed to accommodate specific dietary needs and prevent histamine reactions.

Day 11

- Breakfast: Delightful Morning Fuel: Apricot-Adorned Oatmeal Splash

Introduction: Elevate your mornings with a comforting and nourishing bowl of oatmeal crowned with the sweetness of sliced apricots and a delicate splash of pasteurized milk. This breakfast bowl offers a perfect balance of warmth and fruity freshness to kickstart your day.

Ingredients:
- Oatmeal
- Sliced apricots
- Pasteurized milk

Preparation Method:
Step 1 - Oatmeal Preparation:
- Cook the oatmeal according to package instructions, using water or pasteurized milk for added creaminess.

Step 2 - Sliced Apricots Topping:
- Wash and slice fresh apricots into thin, bite-sized pieces.

Step 3 - Assembling Breakfast:
- Pour the cooked oatmeal into a bowl.
- Top the oatmeal with a generous portion of sliced apricots.
- Add a subtle splash of pasteurized milk over the oatmeal for extra creaminess.

Portion Sizes: Create a balanced breakfast by combining an appropriate portion of oatmeal with a sufficient quantity of sliced apricots. Use a modest amount of pasteurized milk for a delightful finish.

Storage and Handling Tips: Prepare and consume the oatmeal immediately for optimal taste. Store any leftover sliced apricots in an airtight container in the refrigerator and add them to fresh oatmeal later.

Substitutions: Swap pasteurized milk with a dairy-free alternative or yogurt for a creamy twist, catering to specific dietary preferences or lactose intolerance.

Hydration and Beverages: Accompany this breakfast with water, herbal teas, or suitable fruit juices (avoiding citrus) to complement the oatmeal and maintain hydration levels.

Individual Tolerance: Monitor your body's response to oatmeal, apricots, and pasteurized milk. Adjust ingredients or portion sizes as needed to accommodate specific dietary needs and prevent histamine reactions.

- Lunch: Turkey Lettuce Wraps with Creamy Indulgence and Steamed Asparagus Sidekick

Introduction: Enjoy a light yet satisfying lunch featuring succulent turkey slices snugly wrapped in crisp lettuce leaves, adorned with a touch of creamy cream cheese. Accompanied by a nutritious side of steamed asparagus, this meal is a delightful blend of textures and flavors to tantalize your taste buds.

Ingredients:
- Turkey slices
- Lettuce leaves
- Cream cheese
- Asparagus

Preparation Method:
Step 1 - Turkey Lettuce Wraps:
- Lay out the lettuce leaves on a clean surface.
- Place the turkey slices onto the lettuce leaves, spreading a dollop of cream cheese onto each slice.
- Gently wrap the turkey with the lettuce leaves, securing them with toothpicks if needed.

Step 2 - Steamed Asparagus:
- Wash the asparagus spears and trim off the woody ends.
- Steam the asparagus in a steamer basket over boiling water for approximately 4-6 minutes or until tender yet slightly crisp.

Portion Sizes: Prepare a moderate amount of turkey lettuce wraps and serve alongside a suitable portion of steamed asparagus for a balanced lunch.

Storage and Handling Tips: Consume the meal immediately to preserve the freshness and crispness of the lettuce wraps. Store any leftover components separately in airtight containers in the refrigerator for up to 1-2 days.

Substitutions: Substitute cream cheese with a dairy-free alternative or hummus for a different flavor profile or dietary preference.

Hydration and Beverages: Pair this lunch with water, herbal teas, or suitable fruit juices (avoiding citrus) to complement the meal and maintain proper hydration.

Individual Tolerance: Monitor your body's response to turkey, lettuce, cream cheese, and asparagus. Adjust ingredients or portion sizes as needed to accommodate specific dietary needs and prevent histamine reactions.

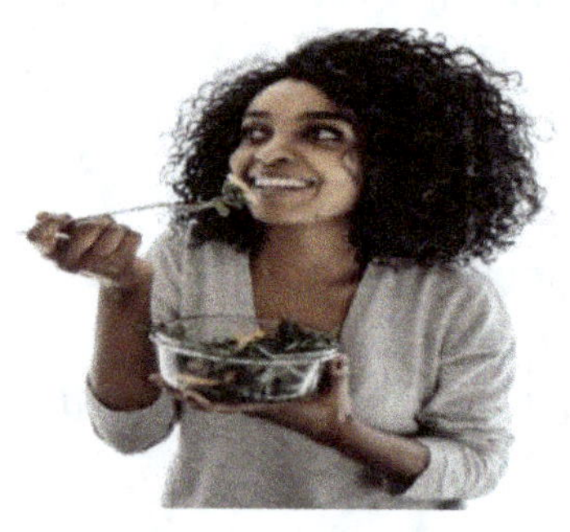

- Dinner: Baked Salmon Brilliance with Sautéed Onions and Velvety Mashed Potatoes

Introduction: Indulge in a delightful dinner featuring succulent baked salmon adorned with sautéed onions, accompanied by a comforting side of velvety mashed potatoes. This dish combines the richness of salmon, the savory appeal of onions, and the comforting warmth of mashed potatoes for a satisfying dining experience.

Ingredients:
- Salmon filet (fresh or frozen)
- Onions
- Potatoes

Preparation Method:
Step 1 - Baked Salmon:
- Preheat the oven to 375°F (190°C).
- Season the salmon filet with your preferred low histamine herbs and spices.
- Place the seasoned salmon on a baking tray lined with parchment paper.
- Bake in the preheated oven for approximately 12-15 minutes or until the salmon is cooked through and flakes easily with a fork.

Step 2 - Sautéed Onions:
- Peel and slice the onions into thin strips.
- Heat a skillet over medium heat and add a touch of oil.

- Sauté the sliced onions until they turn golden brown and caramelized.

Step 3 - Mashed Potatoes:
- Peel and dice the potatoes into chunks.
- Boil the potato chunks in a pot of water until they are tender.
- Drain the water and mash the potatoes using a potato masher. Season as desired.

Portion Sizes: Aim for a suitable portion of baked salmon, a portion of sautéed onions to complement, and an appropriate serving of mashed potatoes for a fulfilling dinner.

Storage and Handling Tips: Enjoy the meal immediately for optimal taste. Store any leftover components separately in airtight containers in the refrigerator for up to 1-2 days.

Substitutions: Consider using another type of low histamine fish based on availability and personal taste. Swap potatoes with a different low histamine root vegetable or cauliflower for a unique twist.

Hydration and Beverages: Accompany this dinner with water, herbal teas, or suitable fruit juices (avoiding citrus) to complement the meal and maintain proper hydration.

Individual Tolerance: Monitor your body's response to salmon, onions, and potatoes. Adjust ingredients or portion sizes as needed to accommodate specific dietary needs and prevent histamine reactions.

Day 12

- Breakfast: Scrambled Yolk Delight with Sautéed Onions and a Peachy Sidekick

Introduction: Start your day on a delightful note with a scrumptious breakfast featuring velvety scrambled egg yolks, savory sautéed onions, and a sweet side of sliced peaches. This breakfast ensemble offers a delightful contrast of flavors to kickstart your morning.

Ingredients:
- Egg yolks
- Onions
- Peaches

Preparation Method:
Step 1 - Scrambled Egg Yolks:
- Crack the eggs and separate the yolks from the whites.
- Whisk the egg yolks gently in a bowl.
- Heat a non-stick skillet over low-medium heat and add a touch of oil or butter.
- Pour the whisked egg yolks into the skillet and gently scramble until they reach the desired consistency.

Step 2 - Sautéed Onions:
- Peel and finely chop the onions.
- Heat a skillet over medium heat, add a touch of oil or butter.
- Sauté the chopped onions until they turn golden brown and caramelized.

Step 3 - Sliced Peaches:
- Wash and slice fresh peaches into thin wedges or slices.

Portion Sizes: Prepare an appropriate amount of scrambled egg yolks, a side of sautéed onions, and a serving of sliced peaches for a satisfying breakfast portion.

Storage and Handling Tips: Consume the breakfast immediately to relish the freshness and flavors. Store any leftover components separately in airtight containers in the refrigerator for up to 1-2 days.

Substitutions: Replace peaches with other low histamine fruits like mangoes or apricots for a varied breakfast experience. Adjust seasonings and herbs for personalized flavor preferences.

Hydration and Beverages: Pair this breakfast with water, herbal teas, or suitable fruit juices (avoiding citrus) to complement the meal and maintain proper hydration.

Individual Tolerance: Monitor your body's response to egg yolks, onions, and peaches. Adapt portion sizes or ingredients if necessary to accommodate specific dietary needs and prevent histamine reactions.

- Lunch: Grilled Chicken Salad Symphony with Cucumber, Beets, and Savory Vinaigrette

Introduction: Relish a refreshing and wholesome lunch featuring tender grilled chicken atop a bed of crisp cucumber and earthy beets, drizzled with a savory vinaigrette made from rich animal fats and herbs. This salad harmoniously blends textures and flavors for a delightful midday meal.

Ingredients:
- Grilled chicken
- Cucumber
- Beets
- Animal fats (for vinaigrette)
- Herbs (for vinaigrette)

Preparation Method:
Step 1 - Grilled Chicken: (Prepare in line with the preferred method from previous recipes.)
- Grill the chicken until it's perfectly cooked and seasoned to taste.

Step 2 - Salad Base:
- Wash and slice the cucumber into rounds or desired shapes.
- Wash, peel, and slice the beets thinly.

Step 3 - Vinaigrette Preparation:
- Mix animal fats (like rendered chicken fat) with a blend of herbs (such as parsley, thyme, or rosemary) to create a savory vinaigrette. Adjust seasoning to taste.

Step 4 - Assembling Salad:
- Arrange the grilled chicken atop a bed of sliced cucumber and beets.
- Drizzle the savory vinaigrette over the salad for an added depth of flavor.

Portion Sizes: Create a balanced lunch by arranging an adequate portion of grilled chicken on the salad bed of cucumber and beets, ensuring a well-rounded meal.

Storage and Handling Tips: Assemble the salad just before consuming for optimal freshness. Store any leftover components separately in airtight containers in the refrigerator for up to 1-2 days.

Substitutions: Replace animal fats with a preferred salad dressing or olive oil-based vinaigrette to suit dietary preferences or restrictions.

Hydration and Beverages: Accompany this salad with water, herbal teas, or suitable fruit juices (avoiding citrus) to complement the meal and maintain proper hydration.

Individual Tolerance: Monitor your body's response to grilled chicken, cucumber, beets, and the vinaigrette. Adjust portion sizes or ingredients as needed to accommodate specific dietary needs and prevent histamine reactions.

- Dinner: Baked Turkey Elegance with Steamed Squash and Rice Harmony

Introduction: Indulge in a wholesome dinner featuring succulent baked turkey breast paired with delicate steamed squash and a side of comforting rice. This meal brings together the succulence of turkey, the tenderness of squash, and the heartiness of rice for a satisfying dining experience.

Ingredients:
- Turkey breast (baked)
- Squash
- Rice

Preparation Method:
Step 1 - Baked Turkey Breast: (Prepare based on preferred method from earlier recipes.)
- Season the turkey breast and bake it until it's cooked through and reaches the desired tenderness.

Step 2 - Steamed Squash:
- Wash and slice the squash into even pieces.
- Steam the sliced squash until it's tender yet retains a slight firmness.

Step 3 - Rice Preparation:
- Cook the rice according to package instructions or your preferred method until it's fluffy and cooked through.

Portion Sizes: Aim for an appropriate serving of baked turkey breast, a side of steamed squash, and a suitable portion of rice for a well-balanced dinner.

Storage and Handling Tips: Consume the meal promptly to relish the flavors and textures. Store any leftovers of individual components in separate airtight containers in the refrigerator for up to 1-2 days.

Substitutions: Replace turkey breast with another low histamine meat or alternative protein source as per dietary preferences or availability. Substitute rice with quinoa or another low histamine grain for a variation.

Hydration and Beverages: Complement this dinner with water, herbal teas, or suitable fruit juices (avoiding citrus) to enhance the dining experience and ensure adequate hydration.

Individual Tolerance: Observe your body's response to turkey, squash, and rice. Adjust portion sizes or ingredients if necessary to suit specific dietary needs and prevent histamine reactions.

Day 13

- Breakfast: Vibrant Morning Smoothie Bursting with Mango, Cranberries, and Apple

Introduction: Start your day on a refreshing note with a delightful fruit smoothie that combines the tropical essence of mango, the tartness of cranberries, and the sweetness of apple. This invigorating blend provides a burst of flavors to energize your morning.

Ingredients:
- Mango
- Cranberries
- Apple

Preparation Method:
Step 1 - Smoothie Creation:
- Peel and chop the mango into chunks.
- Wash the cranberries and apples, removing any seeds or cores.
- Combine the chopped mango, cranberries, and apple in a blender.

- Blend until smooth, adjusting the consistency with water or a suitable juice (avoiding citrus) if needed.

Preferred Cooking Methods: No cooking involved; use fresh fruits to retain their natural freshness and low histamine levels.

Portion Sizes: Aim for a satisfying serving size of the smoothie, ensuring a balanced intake of nutrients without excessive consumption.

Storage and Handling Tips: Enjoy the smoothie immediately after preparation for optimal taste and freshness. Store any leftover smoothie in a sealed container in the refrigerator for a short period, ideally consuming it within a day.

Substitutions: Replace fruits with other low histamine alternatives like blueberries, apricots, or peaches for variety and suitability based on individual preferences or availability.

Hydration and Beverages: Sip on water, herbal teas, or suitable fruit juices (excluding citrus) to complement this invigorating smoothie and maintain proper hydration throughout the day.

Individual Tolerance: Monitor your body's response to mango, cranberries, and apple. Adjust ingredients or portion sizes as necessary to accommodate specific dietary needs and prevent potential histamine reactions.

- Lunch: Wholesome Lunch Delight: Baked Fish, Sautéed Asparagus, and Velvety Mashed Sweet Potatoes

Introduction: Embrace a wholesome lunch featuring succulent baked fish, delicately sautéed asparagus, and a comforting side of mashed sweet potatoes. This meal combines the goodness of fresh fish, vibrant asparagus, and the richness of sweet potatoes for a fulfilling midday experience.

Ingredients:
- Fish (fresh or frozen)
- Asparagus
- Sweet potatoes

Preparation Method:
Step 1 - Baked Fish: (Prepare according to the preferred method from earlier recipes.)
- Season the fish to taste and bake it until it's cooked thoroughly and flaky.

Step 2 - Sautéed Asparagus:
- Wash the asparagus spears and trim off the woody ends.
- Heat a skillet over medium heat, add a touch of oil or butter.

- Sauté the asparagus until they are tender-crisp and lightly browned.

Step 3 - Mashed Sweet Potatoes:
- Wash, peel, and chop the sweet potatoes into evenly sized chunks.
- Boil or steam the sweet potato chunks until they are fork-tender.
- Mash the cooked sweet potatoes and season them with preferred herbs or spices.

Preferred Cooking Methods: Baking the fish preserves its freshness and minimizes histamine accumulation. Sautéing asparagus and boiling/steaming sweet potatoes are recommended to retain their low histamine levels.

Portion Sizes: Create a balanced plate by serving an appropriate portion of baked fish, a side of sautéed asparagus, and a portion of mashed sweet potatoes for a fulfilling lunch.

Storage and Handling Tips: Enjoy the meal immediately for optimal taste and texture. Store any remaining components separately in airtight containers in the refrigerator for a short duration.

Substitutions: Replace fish with another fresh low histamine protein source such as turkey or chicken. Substitute sweet potatoes with other low histamine vegetables like butternut squash for a diverse meal.

Hydration and Beverages: Pair this lunch with water, herbal teas, or suitable fruit juices (avoiding citrus) to complement the flavors and maintain proper hydration.

Individual Tolerance: Monitor your body's response to fish, asparagus, and sweet potatoes. Adjust portion sizes or ingredients as needed to suit specific dietary needs and prevent potential histamine reactions.

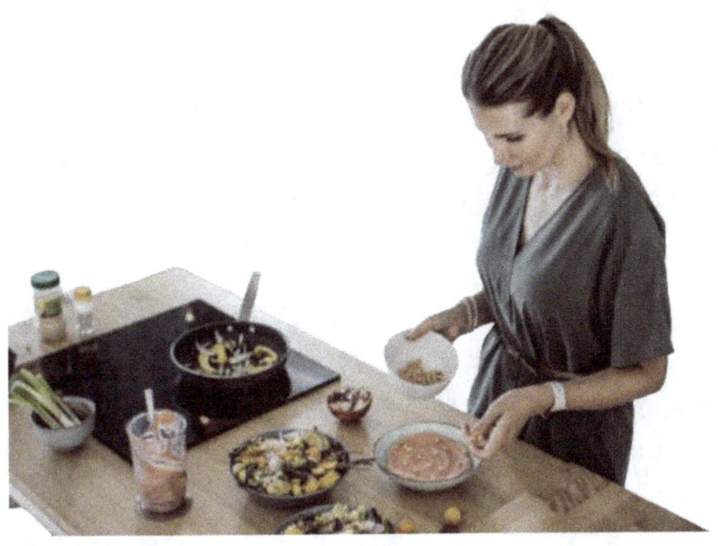

- Dinner: Grilled Chicken Delight with Roasted Beets and Steamed Broccoli Side

Introduction: Enjoy a flavorsome dinner featuring succulent grilled chicken paired with savory roasted beets and a side of vibrant steamed broccoli. This meal amalgamates the tenderness of grilled chicken, the earthy sweetness of roasted beets, and the crispness of broccoli for a satisfying dining experience.

Ingredients:
- Chicken (grilled)
- Beets
- Broccoli

Preparation Method:
Step 1 - Grilled Chicken
- Season the chicken and grill it until it's cooked thoroughly, achieving a delightful charred exterior.

Step 2 - Roasted Beets:
- Wash, peel, and chop the beets into bite-sized pieces.
- Toss the beet pieces with a drizzle of oil and preferred seasonings.
- Roast the seasoned beets in the oven until they are tender and caramelized.

Step 3 - Steamed Broccoli:
- Clean the broccoli and chop it into florets.
- Steam the broccoli until it's tender yet maintains its vibrant green color.

Preferred Cooking Methods: Grilling the chicken maintains its freshness while enhancing its flavor profile. Roasting beets and steaming broccoli are recommended to preserve low histamine levels.

Portion Sizes: Serve an appropriate portion of grilled chicken alongside roasted beets and steamed broccoli for a well-balanced dinner.

Storage and Handling Tips: Consume the meal promptly for optimal taste and texture. Store any leftovers of individual components separately in airtight containers in the refrigerator for a short period.

Substitutions: Swap chicken with another low histamine protein choice like fish or turkey. Substitute beets with carrots or turnips for a varied experience.

Hydration and Beverages: Pair this dinner with water, herbal teas, or suitable fruit juices (excluding citrus) to enhance the meal's flavors and maintain hydration.

Individual Tolerance: Observe your body's response to chicken, beets, and broccoli. Adjust portion sizes or ingredients as needed to accommodate specific dietary needs and prevent potential histamine reactions.

Day 14

- Breakfast: Creamy Oatmeal Bliss with Fresh Cranberries

Introduction: Dive into a comforting breakfast featuring warm oatmeal complemented by the tartness of fresh cranberries and the creamy richness of cream cheese. This delightful combination offers a cozy start to your day with a burst of flavors.

Ingredients:
- Oatmeal
- Fresh cranberries
- Cream cheese

Preparation Method:
Step 1 - Oatmeal Preparation:
- Cook the oatmeal according to package instructions using water or your preferred type of milk until it reaches a smooth and creamy consistency.

Step 2 - Fresh Cranberries:
- Rinse the cranberries thoroughly under running water.

- Gently stir the fresh cranberries into the cooked oatmeal, allowing them to soften slightly with the residual heat.

Step 3 - Cream Cheese Dollop:
- Add a dollop of cream cheese atop the warm oatmeal and cranberries for a creamy and indulgent touch.

Preferred Cooking Methods: Boiling or cooking the oatmeal on the stovetop preserves its texture and flavor. Fresh cranberries and cream cheese add vibrancy and creaminess without the need for cooking.

Portion Sizes: Serve an appropriate portion of oatmeal topped with cranberries and a dollop of cream cheese, ensuring a balanced intake without excessive consumption.

Storage and Handling Tips: Enjoy the oatmeal immediately after preparation to savor its taste and texture fully. Store any leftover oatmeal in an airtight container in the refrigerator for a short duration.

Substitutions: Replace cranberries with other low histamine fruits like sliced peaches or mangoes for variety. Swap cream cheese with a dairy-free alternative or nut butter for a different creamy texture.

Hydration and Beverages: Accompany this breakfast with water, herbal teas, or suitable fruit juices (excluding citrus) to complement the flavors and stay hydrated.

Individual Tolerance: Monitor your body's response to oatmeal, cranberries, and cream cheese. Adjust portion sizes or ingredients as necessary to suit specific dietary needs and avoid potential histamine reactions.

- Lunch: Turkey Stir-Fry Infusion Over Flavorful Rice

Introduction: Relish a lunchtime treat featuring a tantalizing turkey stir-fry infused with the savory goodness of onions, crisp asparagus, and fragrant herbs, served generously over a bed of flavorful rice. This dish melds the succulence of turkey and the aromatic blend of vegetables for a fulfilling and delightful meal.

Ingredients:
- Turkey
- Onions
- Asparagus
- Herbs (from the provided low histamine list)
- Rice

Preparation Method:
Step 1 - Rice Preparation:
- Cook the rice according to package instructions, ensuring it's tender and fluffy. Set it aside.

Step 2 - Turkey Stir-Fry:
- Heat a pan or wok over medium-high heat and add a small amount of oil.

- Sauté the thinly sliced turkey until it's cooked through and slightly browned. Remove from the pan and set it aside.

Step 3 - Veggie Blend:
- In the same pan, add a touch more oil if needed and sauté sliced onions until they're translucent.
- Toss in asparagus spears and continue to stir-fry until they're tender yet crisp.

Step 4 - Herb Infusion:
- Introduce the desired fresh or dried herbs into the pan, infusing the stir-fry with their aromatic essence.

Step 5 - Combination and Serving:
- Reintroduce the cooked turkey to the pan, blending it well with the vegetable medley.
- Serve the flavorful turkey stir-fry over the prepared rice.

Preferred Cooking Methods: Stir-frying the turkey and vegetables swiftly retains their freshness and flavors. Cooking rice separately ensures it's well-cooked without altering its histamine levels.

Portion Sizes: Serve an appropriate portion of turkey stir-fry over rice, aiming for a balanced meal that fulfills but doesn't overindulge.

Storage and Handling Tips: Enjoy the stir-fry immediately to relish its textures and taste. Store any leftovers separately in airtight containers in the refrigerator for a short period.

Substitutions: Exchange turkey with another preferred low histamine protein choice like chicken or fish. Substitute asparagus with bell peppers or broccoli for a diverse stir-fry.

Hydration and Beverages: Accompany this meal with water, herbal teas, or suitable fruit juices (excluding citrus) for a refreshing dining experience.

Individual Tolerance: Monitor your body's reaction to turkey, onions, asparagus, and herbs. Adjust portion sizes or ingredients according to personal dietary requirements to prevent potential histamine-related concerns.

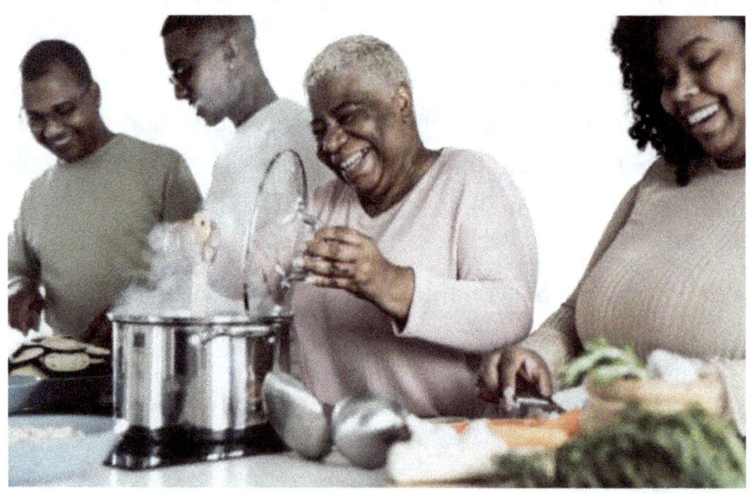

- Dinner: Baked Cod Harmony with Sautéed Squash and Steamed Asparagus

Introduction: Savor a delectable dinner featuring the tender flavors of baked cod accompanied by the delightful combination of sautéed squash and tender steamed asparagus. This dish harmoniously merges the delicate taste of cod with the vibrant, earthy notes of squash and asparagus for a wholesome dining experience.

Ingredients:
- Cod (fresh or frozen)
- Squash
- Asparagus

Preparation Method:
Step 1 - Baked Cod:
- Preheat the oven and prepare a baking dish.
- Place the cod filets in the baking dish, seasoning them with preferred herbs or spices.
- Bake the cod until it's cooked through and flakes easily with a fork.

Step 2 - Sautéed Squash:
- Wash and slice the squash into desired shapes.
- In a separate pan, heat a small amount of oil and sauté the squash until it's tender and lightly golden.

Step 3 - Steamed Asparagus:

- Trim the ends of the asparagus and steam it until it's tender yet retains its vibrant color.

Preferred Cooking Methods: Baking the cod helps maintain its moisture and flavor while avoiding histamine accumulation. Sautéing squash quickly preserves its texture, and steaming asparagus ensures its freshness without altering histamine levels.

Portion Sizes: Serve an appropriate portion of baked cod alongside sautéed squash and steamed asparagus for a well-balanced dinner.

Storage and Handling Tips: Consume the dish promptly to relish its taste and texture. Store any leftover components separately in airtight containers in the refrigerator for a short duration.

Substitutions: Substitute cod with another low histamine fish like haddock or pollock. Replace squash with zucchini or bell peppers for a different flavor profile.

Hydration and Beverages: Pair this delightful dinner with water, herbal teas, or suitable fruit juices (excluding citrus) to complement the flavors and maintain hydration.

Individual Tolerance: Monitor your body's response to cod, squash, and asparagus. Adjust portion sizes or ingredients as necessary to accommodate specific dietary needs and prevent potential histamine reactions.

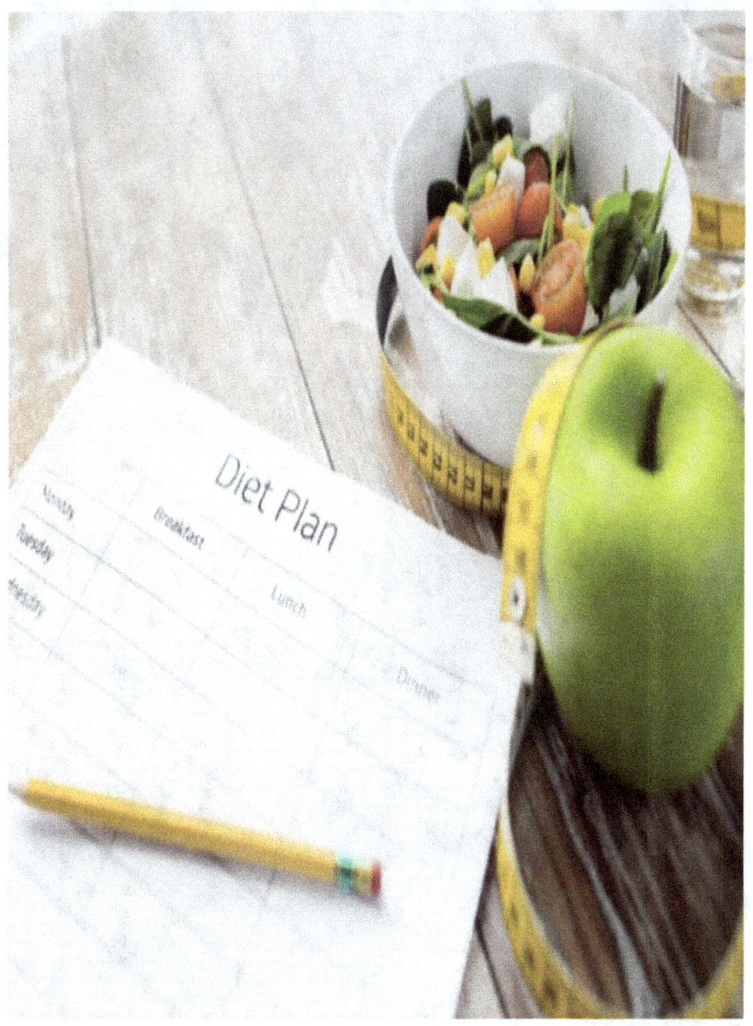

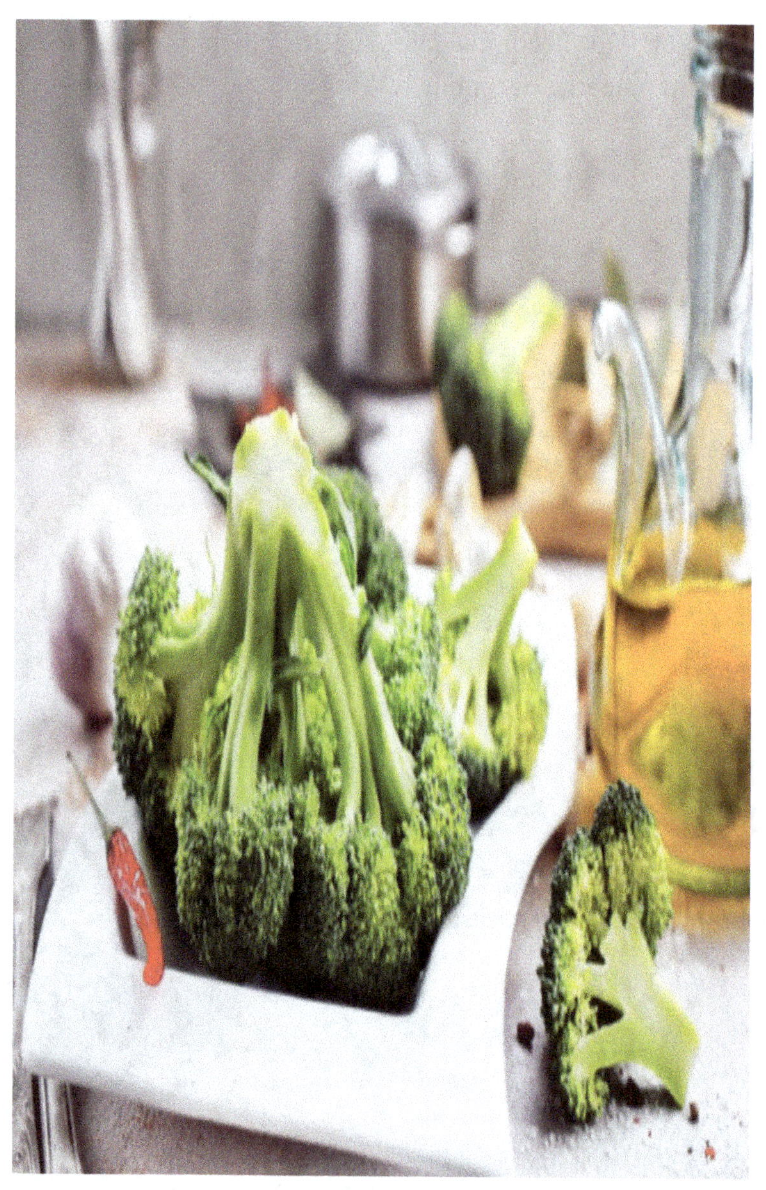

CONCLUSION

Cheers to Your Flavorful Journey!

And just like that, you've reached the end of your 14-day low histamine meal plan! High fives all around for diving headfirst into this flavorful adventure.

Reflecting on Your Journey

Take a moment to pat yourself on the back. Whether you're a seasoned pro at managing histamine intolerance or just dipping your toes into this culinary world, you've taken steps toward nurturing your body and embracing a more mindful approach to eating.

From Meals to Memories

From those cozy breakfast oats to those zesty, low histamine dinners, each meal was a chance to nourish yourself with foods that keep you feeling your best. Remember those delicious blueberries atop your morning oats? They weren't just a sweet treat; they were a nutritious powerhouse!

It's Not Goodbye, It's See You Later

As you bid adieu to this meal plan, remember, it's not goodbye – it's a "see you later." Keep those recipes close, savor those flavors, and let the lessons learned during these

14 days guide you on your ongoing histamine management journey.

Here's to Your Health!

Here's a toast to your well-being! May you continue to explore, experiment, and indulge in foods that make you feel fantastic. And hey, don't forget to stay hydrated, listen to your body, and keep those stress levels in check – they're all part of the recipe for feeling great.

So, as you venture forth, armed with newfound culinary wisdom and a taste for low histamine delights, remember, you've got this! Here's to a future filled with flavorful adventures and a healthy, happy you!

Bon Appétit and keep savoring those delicious moments!

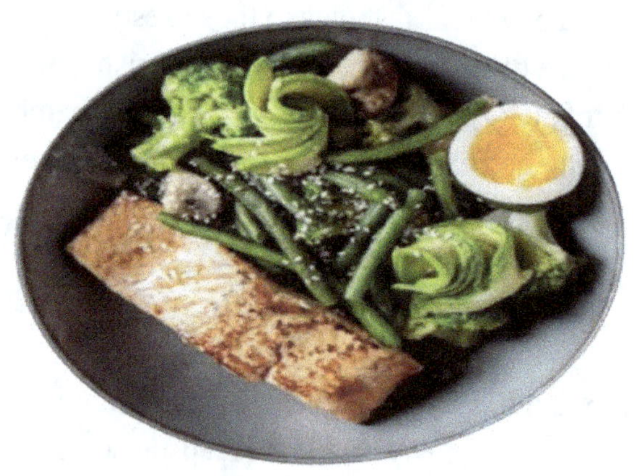

HEY THERE, AMAZING READER!

Thanks a million for taking the time to dive into the "Histamine Intolerance Cookbook." I hope these recipes and insights have added a sprinkle of culinary magic to your life!

Your support means the world to me, and hey, if you loved the journey we took together, how about leaving a review? Your thoughts and feedback not only help others discover this treasure trove but also fuel my passion to whip up even more deliciousness for you.

And hey, sharing is caring, right? If you know someone sailing the seas of histamine intolerance or anyone who could benefit from these culinary wonders, do them a solid and pass on the goodness. Trust me; it might just be the recipe for someone else's happy, symptom-free kitchen adventures!

So, once again, thank you for being a part of this flavorful journey. Let's keep spreading the joy of delicious, low histamine eats together!

Bon Appétit and happy sharing!

BONUS

*Congratulations on grabbing the **"Histamine Intolerance Cookbook"**! As a thank-you treat, you've unlocked a **BONUS**: a delightful collection of 30 FAQs and their witty, oh-so-helpful answers on mastering the low histamine diet.*

Think of it as your personal FAQ cheat sheet - a secret weapon to decode those histamine mysteries and uncover the tastiest, symptom-free culinary adventures!

***Fun Fact:** Did you know histamine isn't just the party pooper causing allergy chaos? It's also a key player in our body's immune response and plays a role in regulating our sleep-wake cycle. Talk about a multitasking molecule!*

So, get ready to dish out those scrumptious low histamine recipes while arming yourself with the wisdom from these FAQs. Let's cook up some flavor-filled, symptom-free magic together!

30 FAQS ON THE LOW HISTAMINE DIET

1. Are there any low histamine substitutes for vinegar in recipes?

 - Lemon juice or apple cider vinegar diluted in water might serve as lower histamine alternatives to vinegar.

2. Can individuals on a low histamine diet consume fermented foods if they're homemade?

 - Homemade fermented foods might have lower histamine levels compared to store-bought versions, but caution and moderation are still advisable.

3. Is there a connection between a low histamine diet and leaky gut syndrome?

 - Some individuals with histamine intolerance believe that following a low histamine diet might help alleviate symptoms associated with leaky gut syndrome, but scientific evidence is limited.

4. Are there specific cooking methods or appliances better suited for low histamine meal preparation?

 - Cooking methods like steaming, baking in parchment paper, or using slow cookers at lower temperatures might help retain nutrients and minimize histamine formation.

5. Can individuals following a low histamine diet use certain supplements to aid in histamine breakdown?

- Supplements like quercetin, vitamin C, or bromelain might help support histamine breakdown, but individual responses can vary.

6. Is it safe to consume leftovers stored in the freezer on a low histamine diet?

- Freezing might help minimize histamine accumulation, but consuming freshly prepared meals is generally recommended over relying solely on frozen leftovers.

7. Are there specific low histamine flours suitable for baking?

- Non-gluten flours like rice flour, coconut flour, or millet flour might be tolerated better than wheat flour by some individuals on a low histamine diet.

8. Can histamine intolerance cause digestive issues beyond typical symptoms like bloating or diarrhea?

- Some individuals with histamine intolerance might experience less common digestive issues like gastroparesis or irritable bowel syndrome (IBS).

9. Are there specific low histamine sweeteners suitable for use in cooking or baking?

- Natural sweeteners like pure maple syrup, honey (if tolerated), or stevia might be low histamine alternatives to processed sugars.

10. Can stress management techniques improve symptoms for individuals with histamine intolerance?

- Stress reduction practices like meditation, yoga, or deep breathing exercises might help alleviate symptoms by minimizing histamine release.

11. Is there a connection between histamine intolerance and hormonal imbalances in women?

- Some women with histamine intolerance report a correlation between hormone fluctuations, especially during menstruation, and increased histamine-related symptoms.

12. What's the role of gut health in managing histamine intolerance?

- Maintaining a healthy gut with probiotics, prebiotics, and a balanced diet might assist in managing histamine intolerance symptoms for some individuals.

13. Are there specific low histamine cooking oils suitable for use in everyday meals?

- Oils like olive oil, coconut oil, or avocado oil are generally well-tolerated and can be used in low histamine meal preparation.

14. Can histamine intolerance affect mental health or mood?

- Some individuals with histamine intolerance might experience mood swings, anxiety, or depression, potentially linked to histamine's impact on neurotransmitters.

15. Is there a connection between histamine intolerance and chronic fatigue syndrome?

- Some individuals with chronic fatigue syndrome report improvements in symptoms by adopting a low histamine diet, but it may vary among individuals.

16. Are there specific herbs or spices that should be avoided on a low histamine diet?

- Certain high histamine herbs and spices like cinnamon, cloves, or paprika might trigger symptoms in sensitive individuals and are best avoided.

17. Can histamine intolerance affect children or infants?

- Histamine intolerance might manifest in children or infants, but diagnosis and management in younger individuals can be challenging and require professional guidance.

18. Are there specific low histamine beverages suitable for hydration other than water?

- Herbal teas like chamomile or rooibos tea, and certain fruit juices like pear or apple juice (avoiding citrus), might serve as low histamine options for hydration.

19. Can individuals with histamine intolerance consume fermented alcoholic beverages like kombucha or kefir?

- Alcoholic beverages that are fermented might significantly increase histamine levels and are generally advised against for those managing histamine intolerance.

20. What's the role of histamine in allergic reactions beyond typical symptoms like sneezing or itching?

- Histamine plays a vital role in anaphylactic reactions, which can involve severe symptoms like difficulty breathing, swelling, or a drop in blood pressure.

21. Can histamine intolerance impact athletic performance or exercise tolerance?

- Some individuals might experience decreased exercise tolerance or heightened fatigue during physical activity due to histamine-related symptoms.

22. Are there specific low histamine snacks suitable for on-the-go consumption?

- Fresh fruits, rice cakes, homemade trail mix with low histamine nuts and seeds, or popcorn might serve as suitable low histamine snacks.

23. Can histamine intolerance be triggered or exacerbated by environmental factors other than allergens?

- Extreme temperatures, pollution, or strong odors might trigger histamine release or worsen symptoms for some individuals.

24. Are there specific low histamine foods that can potentially impact thyroid health?

- Some individuals with thyroid conditions report symptom improvement by incorporating a low histamine diet, but individual responses vary.

25. Can histamine intolerance cause skin issues beyond common symptoms like hives or rashes?

- Histamine intolerance might manifest in less common skin issues like eczema, psoriasis, or flushing.

26. Are there specific low histamine cooking techniques suitable for preserving nutrients in meals?

- Cooking techniques like steaming or baking at moderate temperatures might help retain nutrients while minimizing histamine accumulation.

27. Can histamine intolerance affect oral health or dental issues?

- Some individuals with histamine intolerance might experience oral symptoms like dry mouth, oral ulcers, or gingivitis, potentially linked to histamine's impact on saliva production and immune response.

28. Are there specific low histamine meal planning strategies for individuals with other dietary needs, such as gluten-free or vegetarian diets?

- Individuals with multiple dietary requirements might benefit from planning meals with low histamine ingredients that align with their specific dietary restrictions, seeking guidance if necessary.

29. Can histamine intolerance affect the immune system's response to common illnesses or infections?

- Histamine's role in the immune system might influence an individual's response to infections or illnesses, potentially impacting symptoms or recovery.

30. Is there a connection between histamine intolerance and neurological conditions like migraines or vertigo?

- Some individuals with migraines or vertigo find that managing histamine levels through a low histamine diet might alleviate symptoms, but the relationship varies among individuals.

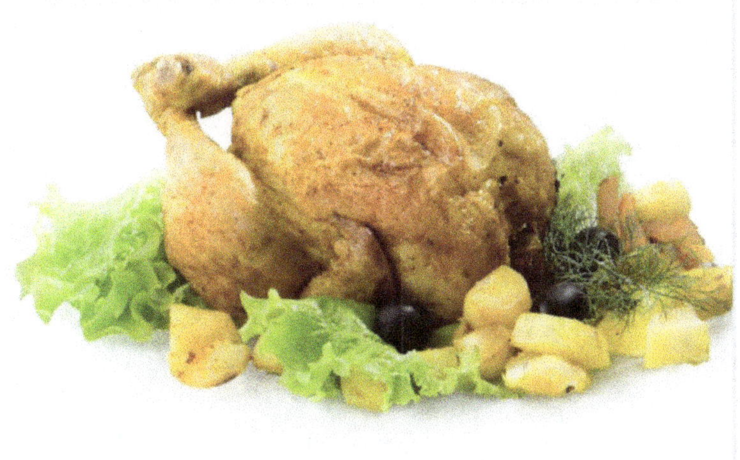

9 798874 001254